THE ESSENTIAL GUIDE TO FOOT AND HAND REFLEXOLOGY

by Ann ers

THE ESSENTIAL GUIDE TO FOOT
AND HAND REFLEXOLOGY by Ann Gillanders
ISBN 0-9511868-5-X (pbk)
ISBN 1-903226 007 (cased)

Text and Illustrations*
copyright ©ANN GILLANDERS 1998

Cover design, book design, illustrations and typesetting by Eleanor Tanner.
Typeface 11 on 13.5 pt Palatino and Helvetica

Prepared for print by
Eleanor Tanner Design, 25 Godfrey Way,
Great Dunmow, Essex CM6 2AY.

Printed and bound in Great Britain
by The Alden Press, Oxford.

Published 1998 by Ann Gillanders.
Reprinted 2000, 2001 and 2002

Acknowledgements
The author would like to express her special thanks to Eleanor Tanner for all the hours spent in the design and artistic editing of this book. And to Margaret Pollock for her indepth understanding of anatomy and physiology and appropriate editing.

* Copyright acknowledgement
The following diagrams are taken from 'The Sourcebook of Medical Illustration' for which the author has permission: the copyright is held by The Medical College of St. Bartholomew's Hospital, London. Figs. 3.1, 6.2, 6.5, 6.6, 6.7, 8.2, 8.3, 8.5, 9.10, 10.2, 10.3, 10.4, 12.2, 13.2 - 13.5, 16.2, 16.3, 18.1 - 18.5, part 20.1, 20.2, 20.3, 22.2, & 32.6.

*GATEWAYS TO HEALTH & HARMONY
WITH REFLEXOLOGY
ISBN 0-9511868-4-1, a companion book to this title, contains detailed CASE HISTORIES and is available from The British School of Reflexology.*

A **Mail Order Catalogue** of Reflexology products and other books by Ann Gillanders is available from **The British School of Reflexology.** A **Register** of qualified practitioners trained by **The British School of Reflexology** and a **Prospectus of Professional Reflexology Training Courses** are also available. *Enquiries to: Ann Gillanders, Principal, The British School of Reflexology, The Holistic Healing Centre, 92 Sheering Road, Old Harlow Essex CM17 0JW* **Telephone 01279 429060 Fax 01279 445234**

Contents

About the author

ANN GILLANDERS is the Principal of **The British School of Reflexology**. Ann and her brother **Tony Porter** were the true pioneers of reflexology some 25 years ago and were responsible for the development of reflexology throughout the United Kingdom. Ann's career has been both extensive and varied, although directed entirely to the fields of medicine and healing. In 1973 she was introduced to reflexology: at that time it was a completely unknown science, and often ridiculed. Ann trained with Dwight Byers, Director of the International Institute of Reflexology, in Florida U.S.A.

After qualifying she established a large practice in Harlow where she still practises today.

In 1979 Ann undertook a teacher-training course with Dwight Byers where she promoted reflexology and set up the United Kingdom side of that Institute, establishing training schools in London, Manchester, Switzerland, Paris and Israel.

In 1986 **The British School of Reflexology** was founded by Ann Gillanders.

In 1989 Ann studied acupresssure and remedial massage with Dr. Louie Chung, Director of the School of Oriental Medicine and obtained a Diploma in both these sciences.

In September 1997, **The British School of Reflexology** opened training schools in both Hong Kong and Japan.

Ann has written and published many books on reflexology. For information on these and other mail order products including books on related subjects, charts and therapy equipment, please contact:

The Holistic Healing Centre, 92 Sheering Road, Old Harlow, Essex CM17 0JW. Telephone 01279 429060 FAX 01279 445234

Introduction

There is a powerful universal energy flowing through the human body. Sometimes referred to as 'chi', or 'the life force', perhaps it should just be called 'love'.

This energy flow cannot be cancelled, destroyed or impeded in any way because it is the very essence of man who centuries ago relied on his intuition, knowledge of roots, herbs and shrubs and sensitivity of touch – he used his hands for healing.

Today, with the rapid progression of drugs and surgery since the end of the war, man is seeking out other more simplistic forms of healing to help heal himself.

As we are all well aware, drugs have an ultimate negative effect on other important functions of the body, in fact many people feel that the side effect of the drug caused them more suffering than the illness for which they were being treated.

Foot and hand reflexology has now been proved to be a very safe and effective way of helping the body to heal itself, and we are able to treat most of the everyday problems which a patient would consult his or her GP about with considerable results.

Touch therapies are growing in popularity, and the one to one communication which reflexology offers has tremendous advantages in stimulating the healing process. For whatever the reasons, we do know that patients treated with reflexology feel better and enjoy a new found mental and physical relaxation. Biological and psychological disorders often leave them after they seek the help of a reflexologist.

I have been involved now for some 25 years in the treatment of patients, the training of therapists throughout the world, writing books and unfolding the mysteries attached to the success of reflexology.

I am sure that in years to come it will be shown that the stimulating of an energy flow, encourages an improvement in nerve and blood supply, a balancing of the body, and an enhancement of relaxation. As we

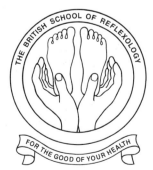

all know, tension is at the seat of disease. Medical doctors today are accepting more and more that the stresses of modern everyday living are responsible for the disorders of the body.

There are over 7,000 nerve endings in each foot. Maybe this fact, more than any other, explains why we feel so much better when our feet are treated and so miserable when our feet are in an uncomfortable state. Corns and calluses have an adverse effect on the body and I am sure we have all experienced a situation when we have walked for too long around a busy town on a hot summer's day in new shoes; at the end of that day we feel ill all over.

I have heard it said that 'the pains in her feet were reflected in her face'.

The purpose of writing this technical training manual is to produce a 'Bible' for the practitioner and a training manual for the student, and to impart to those who have a vested interest in reflexology the vast amount of knowledge and experience that I have attained in my long years involved full time in the development of reflexology.

I still get a tremendous thrill from seeing the benefits that reflexology can achieve in the most chronic situations and the excitement stimulated by our well trained practitioners who go out into the world, develop large practices and further the benefits of reflexology even more.

Good health is a gift and I am sure that eventually the day will come when reflexology will not only be used for treating illness but will also be employed by the public as a way of maintaining good health.

Remember: "Yesterday was the past. Tomorrow's the future. Today is a GIFT and we call it the present."

Ann Gillanders.

How this book is organised

- Chapters 1 to 5 describe reflexology, zone therapy and the guidelines of the feet upon which reflexology is based.
- Chapters 6 to 25 describe the systems of the body and foot reflexology. Each system is fully described and supported with diagrams and is followed by relevant, illustrated practical procedures associated with each system.
- Chapters 26 and 27 describe hand reflexology and relevant practical procedures.
- The full colour foot and hand reflexology charts are to be used in conjunction with the diagrams for practical procedures.
- Subsequent chapters give background information to support and enhance the practice of reflexology.
- Before reading the chapters on practical procedures, study the notes below, which apply to all procedures described. Diagrams on the following page show multiple views of the feet and directions for working.

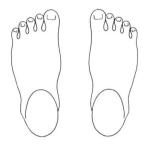

Dorsal view

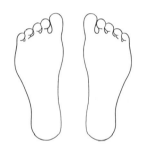

Plantar view

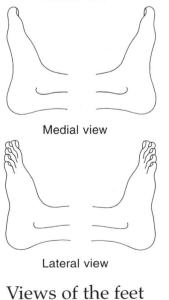

Medial view

Lateral view

Views of the feet

Practical procedures – points to remember:

- It is absolutely essential when working on the feet to adopt the practical procedures in the order they appear in the book.
- It is essential to maintain the habit of working all areas in both directions, exactly in the order indicated in the following chapters where you will find detailed practical instructions on how to work out and identify the way the feet exactly mirror the human body.
- By following the procedures and covering all areas completely, there is no possibility of any reflex area being 'missed'.
- Reflex points are only the size of pinheads!

Right foot
– medial
to lateral

Right foot
– lateral
to medial

Left foot
– medial
to lateral

Left foot
– lateral
to medial

Medial side of feet

Lateral side of feet

Working the feet

Working the right foot – medial to lateral

When starting to work on the right foot you must support the foot in your left hand and work from the medial side to the lateral side of the foot with the right thumb.

Working the right foot – lateral to medial

As you change direction, you must support the right foot with your right hand and, using the left thumb, work back from lateral to medial.

Working the left foot – medial to lateral

When starting to work on the left foot you must support the foot in your right hand and use the left thumb as you work from the medial side to the lateral side of the foot.

Working the left foot – lateral to medial

As you change direction you must then support the left foot with the right hand and work back from the lateral to the medial side with the right thumb.

Working the medial side of the foot

To work the medial side of the foot, hold the foot in an upward direction supporting the lateral side.

Working the lateral side of the foot

When working the lateral side of the foot, hold the foot in an upward direction supporting the medial side.

Supporting the foot

• Support the top of the foot when working above the waist line.
• Support the heel of the foot when working areas below the waist line.

CHAPTER **1** Zones and guidelines

ZONES

Zones are longitudinal lines of energy ascending from the feet to the brain. Reflexology is based on zone therapy. As we apply pressure to the feet, we are working on this basis, stimulating these lines which have a rejuvenating and healing effect on the entire human body.

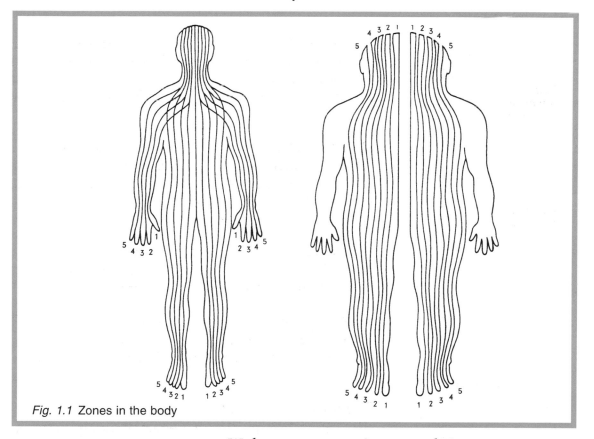

Fig. 1.1 Zones in the body

We have ten zones, five on each foot representing a simple numbering system, with the big toe as Zone 1, the second – Zone 2, the third – Zone 3, the fourth – Zone 4 and the fifth – Zone 5. The fingers link up to the zones in the same way, with the thumb being Zone 1 and the little finger, Zone 5. *See Figures 1.1 and 1.2.*

Zones in the body run from the toes to the brain. There are five zones on either side of the spine.

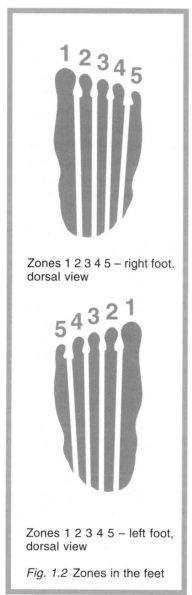

Zones 1 2 3 4 5 – right foot. dorsal view

Zones 1 2 3 4 5 – left foot, dorsal view

Fig. 1.2 Zones in the feet

Zones are distributed through the body like slices. As we work on the plantar or dorsal side of the feet, we are automatically working through the whole of the human body. A sensitivity in any one spot of the foot creates an imbalance in the entire length of that zone. For example, a sensitivity in the right kidney could be the cause of your eye condition, the kidney and eye being in the same zone.

Zone 1 is the most powerful zone in the body because within that zone are many vital functions and parts of the human form: here we have the all important central nervous system, spine and brain and the pituitary gland which is said to be the first gland formed at conception, and often referred to as 'the conductor of the orchestra' and is responsible for all glandular secretions. All this glandular activity is from a little gland just the size of a pea!

Our nose is in Zone 1 and without that important aperture, we would not have the ability to breathe, nor eat as our mouth is also in Zone 1. In Zone 1 we also have the commencement of the solar plexus on the left foot: this nerve complexity lies just behind the stomach and is responsible for many moods and sensitivities. In fact, it really is an emotional barometer – solar plexus means, sun, from the word solar, and plexus means a network of nerves.

Our naval is in Zone 1 and this denotes the important link with the placenta and foetus prior to birth – the umbilical cord joining the two and delivering life giving sustenance to the foetus at the same time as removing damaging impurities.

Our reproductive organs are in Zone 1 and are essential for procreation.

When working on people's feet you will find that the first zone is always the most sensitive.

Many sensitivities in this area are caused by back conditions.

The principle of reflexology is to find out and work out the sensitive spots in the feet by an alternating pressure of thumb and sometimes the index fingers on all parts of the foot.

Refinement of the pressure and consistent control is of great importance in achieving a result. All too frequently I hear of people having treatment and getting absolutely no results whatsoever. When treated by a properly qualified practitioner, they are then quite amazed at the outstanding and quick improvement they get in their health problem.

What is a stimulus?

It is any agent or factor which evokes functional reaction in tissues, even inducing a physiological change. In our work, stimulus means contact and pressure which initiates an impulse of a message transmitted through nerve fibres. The pressure applied to a nerve ending constitutes a stimulus.

This stimulus sets in motion a nerve impulse, an electro-chemical impulse which effects a change in nervous processes. Nerve impulses travel at the rate of about 270 miles per hour, whilst electricity travels at the speed of light.

Our bodies are an electro-chemical plant which are in motion throughout the day and night.

Obstructions in the energy lines

The importance of energy lines

Reflexology teaches that every organ and gland depends on its survival by this ability to contract and relax. When an obstacle is placed in the energy channel, as when acid crystals, wastes or unused calcium deposits form on the delicate nerve endings of the feet, the energy flow is impeded and the organ it serves is then adversely affected.

Obstructions in the energy lines and fields register pain and in certain conditions create limitations in motion and functions; for example a stiff neck or a painful back. Energy blockage also interferes with blood circulation and this is usually first noticed in the extremities. Hands may become stiff, cold and often painful. Waste products accumulate at the lowest point of gravity, which can be distinctly felt under the thumb and fingers as you work on the feet.

There is no substitute for the human hand. No

machine can give you this information, and that is why I am totally against all forms of electrical stimulating machines and devices to assist in the treatment of reflexology.

We have far too many machines in our modern, everyday life, so it is vital that we now reach back to the natural ways of healing, and use our hands – hands were meant for healing.

THE GUIDELINES OF THE FEET

Apart from the study of zones, we need to understand the guideline principle of the feet and their relativity to all parts of the body. You cannot learn or administer reflexology without an understanding of these lines.

If you consider that the feet are really nothing less than the mirror of the body. They are miraculous, structural masterpieces, exquisitely and beautifully designed, perfectly coordinating many components. Among these components are tissue, 26 bones, 100 ligaments, 20 muscles and an intricate network of nerves and blood vessels. These marvellous structures also reflect totally our state of health.

The condition of our feet and the way we use them reveals our physical and mental state and influences not only their own performance but the functioning of our mind and body as well.

Likewise how we treat our feet influences our mental and physical health: it is a two-way street – a reciprocal relationship.

Guidelines are quite easily identified by certain outstanding features of the feet and are shown in *Figure 1.3.*

1 The diaphragm line

The diaphragm line is found under the bases of the metatarsals. A distinguishing feature is that the colour of the skin on the metatarsal area is quite remarkably different from the underside of the instep. The darker skin is above our diaphragm line and the lighter skin below, so there is almost an identifying line, as if nature intended to help.

The importance of guidelines

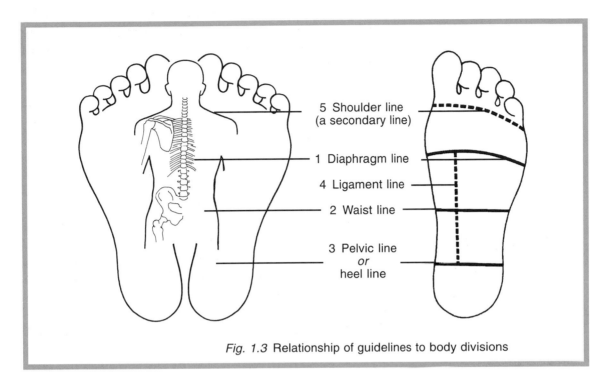

5 Shoulder line
(a secondary line)

1 Diaphragm line

4 Ligament line

2 Waist line

3 Pelvic line
or
heel line

Fig. 1.3 Relationship of guidelines to body divisions

2 The waist line

The waist line is found by running your finger along the lateral side of the foot and feeling a small bony protrusion about midway. When we find this protrusion we then draw a line across the foot; this area is normally in the narrowest part of the foot.

3 The pelvic line

The pelvic line (sometimes called the heel line) is found by drawing an imaginary line from the ankle bones on either side of the foot and crossing over the base of the heel.

4 The ligament line

The ligament line is the ascending line which is on the plantar ligament, that taught elastic-like structure that you can feel if you retract your big toe. Upon this tendon we draw our ligament line.

5 The shoulder line

The shoulder line is found just below the bases of the toes and we refer to this as a secondary line.

Physical
characteristics and
problems reflected in
the feet

The feet and physical characteristics

It is interesting to understand how the feet do reflect our body shape and size.

If you are a tall slim person you will have long slim feet, with slender toes. If you are slim with narrow shoulders, the width of the area from the inside to the outside of the diaphragm line will be narrow.

Your hands too, resemble the shape of your feet. You will not find a person with long slim feet with short fat hands!!

The feet and physical problems

As the area to the cervical spine is found on the medial side of the foot, i.e. at the edge of the big toe, a protrusion on the toe joint in this area, which would be called a bunion, could create a neck condition.

Those who suffer from flat feet are more likely to be troubled with aches, pains and stiffness in the lumbar spine.

Any deep seated corns or calluses can interfere with the energy flow and cause inflammation and congestion in the part of the body that the reflexes are within.

Hard skin that builds up on the lateral sides of the feet, under the fifth toe which reflects the shoulder area can cause tension and pain in the shoulder joint, often called 'a frozen shoulder'.

Consultation with a chiropodist to remove hard skin and deal with corns and calluses prior to commencing reflexology treatment sessions is highly recommended.

CHAPTER 2 Body systems and reflex areas

The human body like that of every other living creature has two prime biological functions – to heal itself and to reproduce and ensure the survival of its offspring.

However, these are only possible when all the bodily functioning works efficiently, effectively and in total harmony. You cannot treat each system of the body as a separate entity: one doctor to treat the respiratory system; the other, the circulatory; the other, the renal function, and so on. Diseases and imbalances in one part of the body ultimately affect all functioning.

In this book we are going to have the opportunity of learning about the human body, understanding the functioning of all the systems and relating this study to reflexology. It is absolutely essential when embarking on a career as a reflexologist to know how the body works, where the reflexes to every organ, function, gland and structure reside in the feet, and also have a knowledge of disease and disharmony, plus an understanding of drugs and their effect upon the body.

1 The digestive system

THE ALIMENTARY CANAL is the system of digestion from the mouth to the rectum. The 9 metres (30 ft) of tubing between the mouth and anus has a complex range of functions: it is needed to eliminate waste products, store and digest food and produce vitamins. In order to have a healthy digestive system, efficient functioning of the immune and nervous systems is necessary.

Emotional upsets have a detrimental effect on our digestive system.

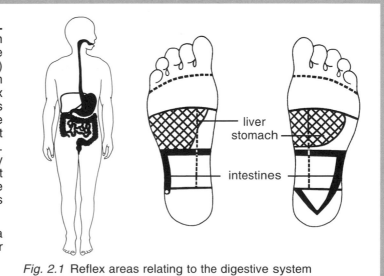

Fig. 2.1 Reflex areas relating to the digestive system

liver
stomach
intestines

2 The respiratory system

THE RESPIRATORY TRACT which relies on proper functioning of the muscles of respiration, carries air in and out of our lungs where the gases oxygen and carbon dioxide are exchanged during respiration.

As we inhale air we also take into our systems dirt and other foreign particles, a variety of chemicals, bacteria, and viruses all of which are threats to our health, but our body's defence mechanisms deal with these invaders.

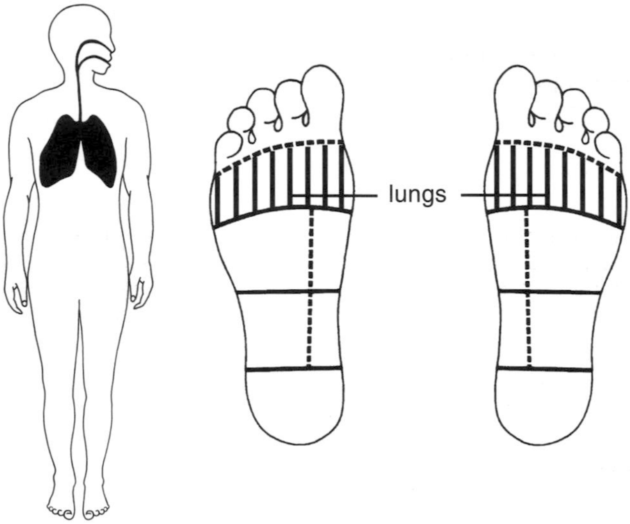

lungs

Fig. 2.2 Reflex areas relating to the respiratory system

3 The circulatory system

THE HEART is a very efficient pump and a tireless muscle. It pumps blood through a vast complex of blood vessels which bring oxygen and nourishment to the cells of the body.

The heart is richly supplied with nerves, blood vessels and lymph vessels.

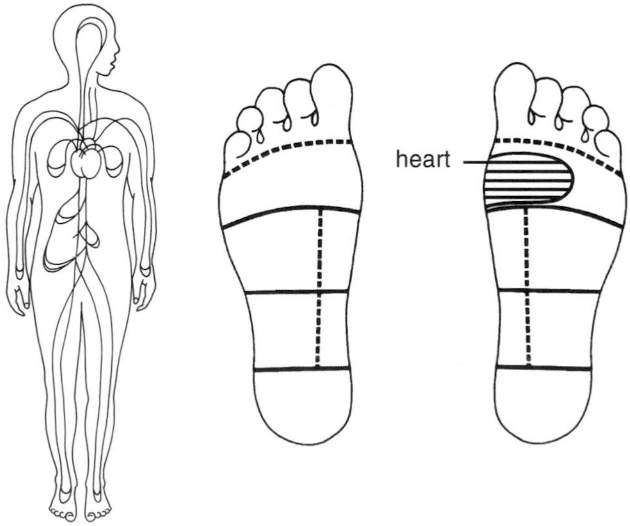

heart

Fig. 2.3 Reflex areas relating to the circulatory system

4 The endocrine system

THE ENDOCRINE SYSTEM consists of tissues and glands which secrete chemical messengers called hormones.

Hormones are released into the surrounding tissues and then diffuse into capillaries and are transported by blood to target tissues.

Hormones regulate growth, reproduction, salt and fluid balance, use of nutrients, metabolic rate and coping with stress.

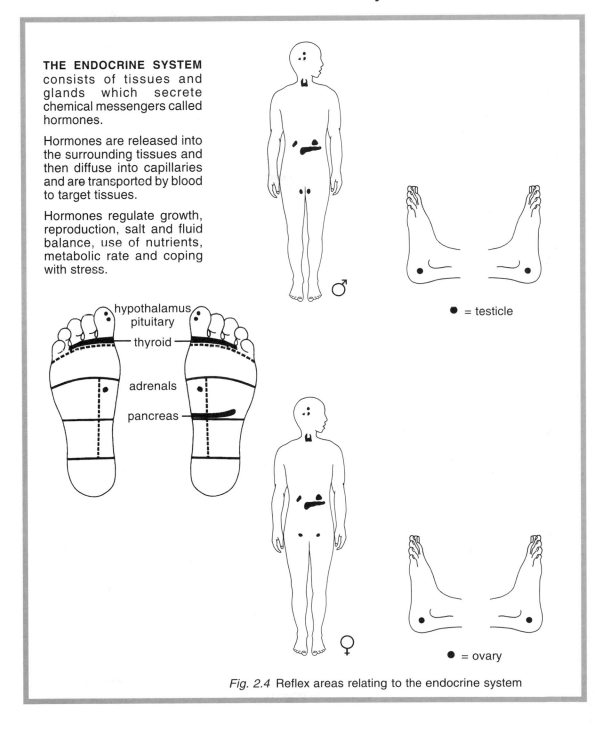

hypothalamus
pituitary
thyroid
adrenals
pancreas

● = testicle

● = ovary

Fig. 2.4 Reflex areas relating to the endocrine system

5 The nervous system

THE BRAIN

All our body movements are controlled by the brain which is the seat of both creativity and consciousness. Through the spinal cord and pairs of nerves arising out of the brain and spine, all bodily movements and functions are conducted.

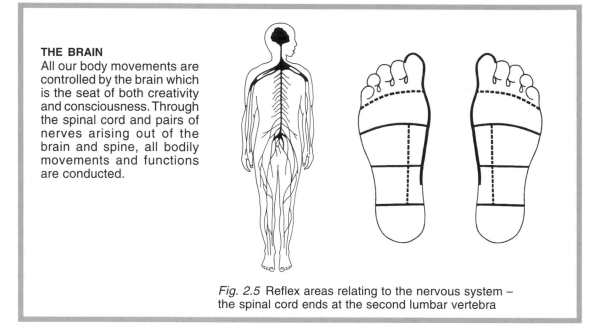

Fig. 2.5 Reflex areas relating to the nervous system – the spinal cord ends at the second lumbar vertebra

6 The muscular system

THE MUSCULAR SYSTEM

Skeletal muscles make up about half the body's bulk. Working with the skeleton, muscles generate the energy to move, make intricate and precise hand movements, and lift heavy objects.

The heart, a very efficient pump, has specialised muscle fibres and pushes blood through a continuous network of blood vessels.

The activity of smooth muscles is important for the functioning of our digestive, respiratory, urinary and reproductive systems.

Muscles rely on a healthy nerve and blood supply.

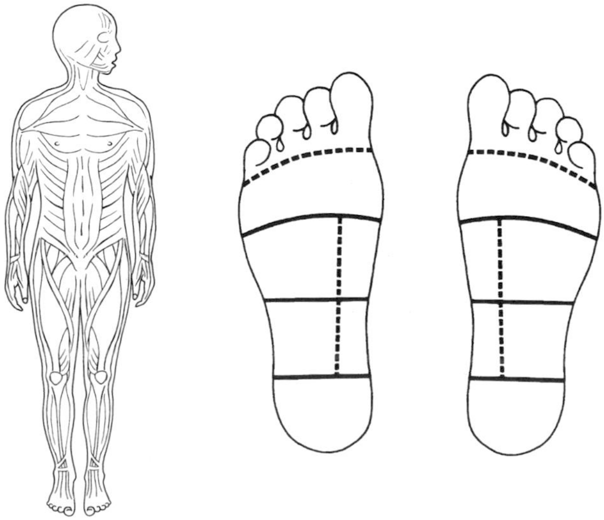

Fig. 2.6 As muscles are within the entire body it is not possible to identify these

7 The lymphatic system

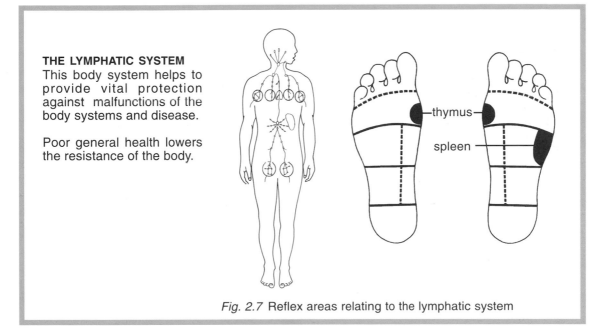

THE LYMPHATIC SYSTEM
This body system helps to provide vital protection against malfunctions of the body systems and disease.

Poor general health lowers the resistance of the body.

Fig. 2.7 Reflex areas relating to the lymphatic system

8 The urinary system

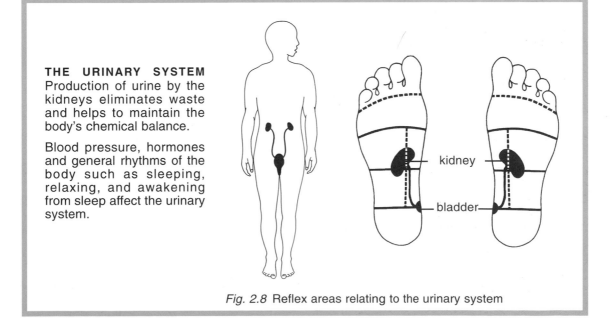

THE URINARY SYSTEM
Production of urine by the kidneys eliminates waste and helps to maintain the body's chemical balance.

Blood pressure, hormones and general rhythms of the body such as sleeping, relaxing, and awakening from sleep affect the urinary system.

Fig. 2.8 Reflex areas relating to the urinary system

9 The reproductive system

THE REPRODUCTIVE SYSTEM

Unlike other bodily systems, the reproductive system in the female functions for only part of the human life span. Although small compared with other systems of the body, its intricate balance and ability to create life is one of life's greatest miracles.

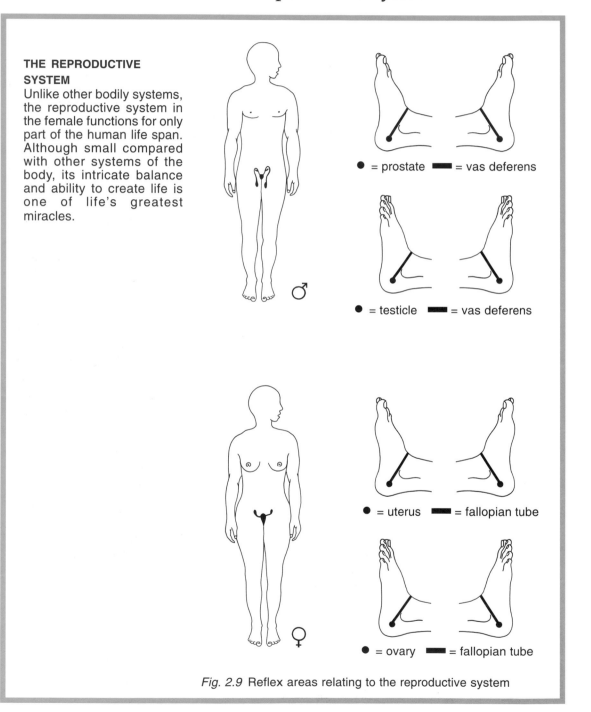

● = prostate ▬ = vas deferens

● = testicle ▬ = vas deferens

● = uterus ▬ = fallopian tube

● = ovary ▬ = fallopian tube

Fig. 2.9 Reflex areas relating to the reproductive system

CHAPTER **3** Cells, tissues and skin

CELLS

The cell is the fundamental unit of life. It is the smallest structure of the human body, capable of performing all the processes that define life, including movement, our respiratory function, digestion, and reproduction.

Cells are called the building blocks out of which all life evolves. We are made of many cells of different shapes and sizes: cells are so minute that most are microscopic and invisible to the human eye. The female sex cell, the largest cell in the human body, is still only the size of the full stop at the end of this paragraph.

The jelly-like material of the cell is called cytopalsm and is bounded by a plasma membrane. The plasma membrane protects the cell and regulates the passage of materials into and out of the cell.

How amazing to understand that when the cell which becomes the embryo in the uterus, divides and multiplies to create a unique individual, everything about you as a person is decided: your approximate height, the colour of your eyes and hair and the unfortunate genetic weaknesses that are carried on from generation to generation by the influence of our cellular make-up.

The nucleus of every cell contains 46 chromosomes, each is a long coiled molecule of DNA and together they contain about 100,000 genes. Every gene is a minute segment of DNA that controls cellular function by governing the synthesis or manufacture of protein.

We not only need proteins for growth and energy, but also for directing specific chemical functions in the body, such as muscle, hair and skin: others carry haemoglobin, and antibodies.

1 Cell structure

The cell contains a fluid called cytoplasm and organelles or cytoplasmic structures with special functions, e.g.

The nucleus

The nucleus is the control centre of the cell and is surrounded by a membrane which appears darker than the surrounding cytoplasm. It contains chromatin which forms chromosomes during cell division.

Mitochondria are concerned with releasing energy from fuel molecules. This process is called cellular respiration.

Endoplasmic reticulum is a system concerned with enzymes, chemical activity, protein manufacture and transport.

Golgi-apparatus produces glycoproteins – mucin required in secretions, secretory enzymes, transports and stores lipids.

Cilia are tiny hairlike organelles projecting from the surfaces of many cells, to help move materials outside the cells, e.g. the cells lining the respiratory passages.

2 Aggregation of living material

Tissue

A group of cells having similar structure and function e.g. muscle and nerve tissue.

Organ

A collection of different tissues grouped together to form an organ which usually has a single function, e.g. stomach made of involuntary muscle, blood, nerves, epithelium, all performing the function of digestion in the first part of the alimentary canal – the gut.

Body system

A group of organs associated together to perform a single overall function e.g. alimentary canal combining together with buccal cavity, oesophagus, stomach, small intestine, large intestine and associated glands i.e. the liver, gall bladder and pancreas.

Organism

The single individual (us) of a species made up of a number of body systems e.g. blood, nervous, muscular, skeletal and digestive. Every cell in the body has a nucleus with the exception of mature red blood cells.

TISSUES

The tissues of the body consist of large numbers of cells. There are four main types of tissue: epithelial tissue or epithelium, connective tissue, muscle tissue and nervous tissue.

1 Epithelial tissue

This is also called epithelium and protects the body by covering all of its free surfaces and lining its cavities. The functions of epithelial tissue is to protect, absorb and secrete.

Epithelial tissue lines our respiratory passages. The cells here are equipped with cilia that beat mucus containing trapped dirt and particles away from the lungs. The taste buds in our mouth consist of epithelium: also our kidney tubules.

2 Connective tissue

This tissue is the packaging between organs of the body and, as it says, connects one part of the body to the other. It also supports and protects the body.

Connective tissue cells are separated by a thick gel which has microscopic fibres throughout. There are three types of connective tissue fibres:

Collagen fibres are the most numerous and contain proteins. These fibres give great strength to structures.

Fine reticular fibres give support to many tissues and organs, e.g. kidneys, brain and lymph nodes.

Elastic fibres are an important part of structures which must stretch, e.g. air sacs and arteries.

The main types of connective tissue are:

Connective tissue proper joins body structures, fills spaces between body parts and acts as a reservoir for water and salt.

Adipose (fat) tissue consists of fat cells which make up 20 to 25 per cent of our body weight. It therefore acts as an insulator. We tend to carry an excess of adipose tissue on our buttocks, thighs, abdomen, breasts and upper arms, if we have a tendency to obesity.

Blood, lymph and tissues that produce blood cells.

Lymphoid tissue
This is found in lymphatic tissues, i.e. the spleen, lymph nodes, the tonsils and adenoids, the appendix and walls of the intestine.

Cartilage
A firm type of connective tissue reinforced by collagen and elastic fibres. There are three types of cartilage: hyaline, fibrocartilage and elastic fibrocartilage.

i) Hyaline cartilage is found on the surface of the parts of the bones which form joints, forms the costal cartilage which connects the ribs to the sternum, and forms part of the larynx, bronchi and trachea.

ii) Fibrocartilage is found between the vertebrae in the form of intervetebral discs.

iii) Elastic cartilage forms the pinna or lobe of the ear, the middle part of a blood vessel and the flap of cartilage which covers the trachea to prevent food going down into our airway, called the epiglottis.

Bone
This is a connective tissue which also produces blood cells. The skeleton provides support, protection and, together with muscles, moves parts of the body.

3 Muscle tissue

Muscle tissue is composed of cells specialized to contract. There are three types of muscle tissue: smooth (involuntary) muscle, skeletal (voluntary) muscle and cardiac muscle which is also considered an involuntary type of muscle.

Smooth muscle
This type of muscle occurs in internal organs and causes involuntary muscle movement.

Skeletal muscle
Skeletal muscle has a striated appearance and is voluntarily controlled. It comprises the bulk of the body's muscle system and is attached to the skeleton.

Cardiac muscle
This muscle is found in the wall of the heart, has striations and is controlled involuntarily.

4 Nervous tissue

Two types of cells are found in the nervous system:

Neurones

They transmit and receive information.

Glial cells

These cells support and nourish neurones.

SKIN

The skin is the largest organ in the body and is capable of self repairing rapidly and effectively. The skin contains many sensory receptors that detect touch, pressure, heat, cold and pain; an awareness is felt of even the lightest touch.

The appearance of a person's skin often gives accurate indicators of their general health.

Most irritations on the skin's surface are caused by irritations within the physical body and the cause for skin troubles, i.e. eczema, boils and acne, and various allergic rashes need to be tackled by treating the physical body – looking for the cause within the body, not without.

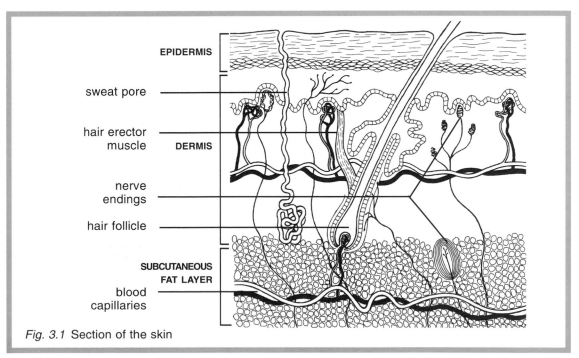

EPIDERMIS

sweat pore

hair erector muscle   DERMIS

nerve endings

hair follicle

SUBCUTANEOUS FAT LAYER

blood capillaries

Fig. 3.1 Section of the skin

1 Skin structure

The skin comprises two main layers: the outer consists of epithelial tissue, layers of skin cells which are near to the surface involved with protection, absorption and secretion and the inner dermis comprised of fibrous and elastic tissue, blood vessels, sweat glands, nerve fibres and hair follicles. Beneath the skin is an underlying subcutaneous layer. *See Figure 3.1.*

2 Skin characteristics

The skin is elastic as well as being protective and is able to stretch to quite enormous proportions if needed, as in the case of pregnancy, and then return to its normal proportions very rapidly.

Our skin eliminates large quantities of fluids in the form of perspiration daily, and although so porous, we still do not drown when we swim in the sea – the oily secretions eliminated by the sebaceous glands keep our skin soft and pliable.

The erector muscles of hair contract when we are cold and these create our 'goose pimples'.

The sensory nerve endings present in the dermis are stimulated by touch, pressure, pain and temperature.

The rapid action needed if we place our hand or finger on a hot surface, is called the reflex action.

CHAPTER 4

Your feet – the mirror of your body

The feet are really nothing less than the mirror of the body. The feet are miraculous structural masterpieces, exquisitely and beautifully designed, perfectly co-ordinating many components. Among the components are muscles, tissues, 26 bones, 100 ligaments, 20 muscles and an intricate network of nerves and blood vessels. These marvellous structures also reflect totally our state of health. *See Figure 4.1.*

The condition of our feet and the way we use them reveals our physical and mental state and influences not only their own performance but the functioning of our mind and body as well.

Likewise, how we treat our feet influences our mental and physical health. It is a two-way street: a reciprocal relationship.

FOOT PROBLEMS

Abuse of the feet and the consequent foot misalignments which cause blisters, bunions, calluses and corns, often cause, in turn, general fatigue and bodily aches

Conversely, systemic or general body disorders, such as rheumatoid arthritis, diabetes, multiple sclerosis and some types of heart disease, show up first in the feet, causing them to hurt some time before the malfunctioning organs have exhibited other symptoms.

Foot pain can indeed camouflage serious diseases, so foot discomfort of any kind demands immediate attention, not only to the foot but to the rest of the body. What may appear to be merely a foot problem could in fact be a symptom of a systemic disease. Medical statistics reveal that two out of three people are plagued with one or more foot problems, so let's look at some of them.

1 Athlete's foot

Although not a disease in itself, athlete's foot represents an entire set of symptoms – scaling between the toes,

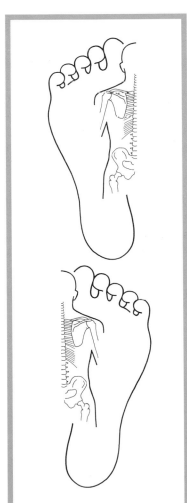

Fig. 4.1 The shape of the body reflected in the shape of the feet

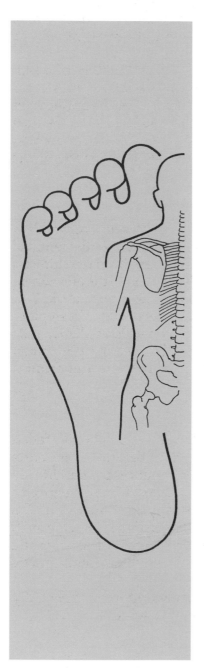

an itching sensation and a softening of the flesh are the most common of them. It may initially be the result of a fungus, but if it becomes chronic roughening of the skin can follow. Known technically as hyperkerato-mycosis, which is a thickening and hardening of the external layer of the skin, athlete's foot occurs more frequently in men than women; it may be a local problem; it can also be the result of an allergy, a drug overdose or sunburn.

Naturopathic doctors believe that athlete's foot is exacerbated by the body's poor elimination of waste; that is, the skin, lungs, bowel and kidney are not performing their eliminating responsibility very efficiently. The feet are then used as an area of elimination and through the perspiration which is normally heavily made up of a highly proteinous material, the virus which creates athlete's foot thrives in abundance. Often attention to the body's eliminating processes in the form of a fast, extra exercise, hot and cold showers, and body scrubs, gives the body a chance to eliminate its waste through the proper channels, and allows the condition to disappear.

2 Bunions

Bunions are another foot problem, the predisposition to which might be inherited, but we do know that a bunion can develop from poorly fitted shoes. In some, but not in all cases the 'bursa' or sac over the joint of the big toe becomes inflamed and swollen, sometimes twisting the big toe under the two next to it. When working on the feet of a person with such a condition and for whom it is painful, you must work on the corresponding place on the hand. Pressure must not be applied to painful swollen areas.

3 Corns and calluses

It is estimated that millions of people suffer from corns and calluses. They can be the result of friction, abnormal foot structure, systemic problems, or even arise through imbalance of mental or emotional upsets. A chiropodist or podiatrist will usually prescribe

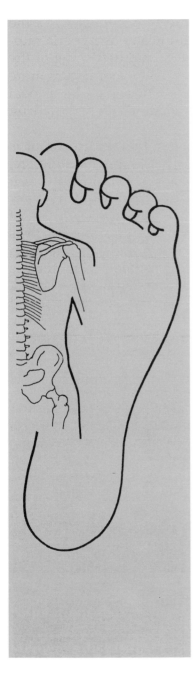

salicylic acid plasters to remove corns and calluses.

Castor oil rubbed twice daily into the affected area softens the corn or callus so that it can eventually be peeled off with the fingers.

Other home remedies are the application of a thin slice of lemon fastened with a sticking plaster or adhesive tape and left for the night, or the application of a piece of cotton dipped in witch hazel to the area over night. After a number of applications over a period of days the skin usually softens enough to remove the corns and calluses gradually.

4 Verrucae

A friend of mine, who is a very good chiropodist, informs me that a good first aid remedy for the removal of a verrucae is to cut a small square from the skin of a banana, place the inside of the skin on to the area where the verrucae is situated and cover it with a piece of sticking plaster. Repeat and replace with a fresh piece daily and within a week the verrucae evidently falls out. I certainly think this would be worth trying if you or somebody in your family is suffering from a verrucae.

5 Fallen arches

Many people are born with a predisposition to fallen arches but many never suffer from them. Arch supports may be helpful in certain circumstances but specifically designed exercises are preferable. It is interesting to note that through the centuries superstitions or myths have developed about the arches of the feet. One such myth is that high arches are a sign of aristocratic descent. Low arches may be an ethnic characteristic and yet cause no pain.

It is said that strong arches are important for healthy feet and for good support of our spine.

6 Rheumatoid arthritis

In its early stage, rheumatoid arthritis may appear as pain, stiffness, or swelling of the joints of the feet. Tiny lumps beneath the skin known as subcutaneous nodules may appear as early warning signs of this serious ailment. You can feel these nodules because it may cause discomfort if pressure is exerted too enthusiastically, particularly during the first reflexology treatment session. When the disease has reached the degenerative, chronic stage, deformities such as hammer toes and bony spurs may appear.

7 Gout

Appearing more frequently in men than in women. It is possible to be genetically predisposed to this condition.

Its appearance is often marked by a sudden change in the big toe which becomes shiny, swollen, inflamed and extremely painful. This initial point of irritation is usually the metatarsophalangeal joint, but other joints in the feet may also be affected. While at first, perhaps mistakenly, it is viewed as a local problem, eventually gout comes to be known for what it is.

Gout is caused by a disturbance in the uric acid metabolism which results in levels in the blood becoming excessive. Because of the build-up of waste products in the system, insoluble uric acid salts accumulate in the blood around the joints and in the tissues in the form of crystalline deposits which one can feel when they are pressed.

8 Cardiovascular diseases

These affect the heart and circulatory system and may cause pain, swelling and a burning sensation in the feet if the blood circulation is impaired.

9 Arteriosclerosis

This is the hardening and thickening of the arteries, which seriously reduces blood flow, with the consequent loss of oxygen to the tissues of the feet and removal of deoxygenated blood. This leads to poor gaseous interchange in the tissues. Difficulty in walking, pain when the feet are at rest, ulcers and infections, loss of hair on the legs, and thickening of the nails, particularly on the big toes, are all clues to the presence of this disorder.

10 Other disorders

Swelling and oedema in the feet and legs can be caused by heart inadequacy. Body fluids then accumulate in the extremities since they are restricted in their flow. An early symptom of diabetes is often a numbness and tingling sensation in the feet. Ulcers may develop on the soles and, if infections occur, they heal very slowly.

Symptoms of neurological problems or nerve disorders, even brain lesions, can appear in the feet in the form of lack of coordination and muscle weakness.

Care of the feet

If you give your feet the kind of care they deserve, the entire system will benefit from mental ease. Here are some tips on the proper care of the feet.

• **Insist on wearing shoes about 1.3 cm (half an inch) longer than your feet and make sure you get the correct width.**

• **Buy shoes in the afternoon; one's feet expand during the day, particularly in hot weather.**

• **Do not wear shoes that are made of synthetic materials: leather shoes or fitted sandals are the best.**

• **If you wear socks they should be wool or cotton and, again, 1.3 cm (half an inch) longer than your feet.**

• **After bathing dry the feet carefully between the toes and use some form of penetrating foot cream.**

• **Cider vinegar is an excellent antiseptic preparation for the feet. All you need is about two tablespoons of cider vinegar in a litre of warm water in which to soak your feet and it will have excellent remedial benefits.**

• **Do not wear tight fitting bands at the top of stockings as these restrict your circulation.**

• **Walking is the best form of exercise.**

Feet and posture

Two important jobs the feet perform are supporting and maintaining one's posture and propelling the body into whichever direction one desires. The big toe is responsible for helping to control balance, along with the intrinsic muscles of the foot. It is estimated that the force to which each foot is subjected during a single day is equivalent to approximately 600 tons for a 68 kilo (150 pound) person.

Did you also realise that within a lifetime the average person walks to the moon and back?

Reflexology's role

Everyone who experiences reflexology can benefit from it, but not all will recover completely. No matter what may be done in terms of pressure therapy, some people will continue to eat the wrong food, drink the wrong beverages, refuse to give up smoking, drinking or taking drugs.

These people refuse to alter their mental attitudes about themselves, and the world about them, preferring to put the responsibility for their ill health into the hands of their local doctor, who they hope, by some magical pill or potion, will give them back their health and energy without any effort being made by themselves to change anything.

Reflexology induces mental and physical relaxation in the body, restores proper circulation and nerve supply and most important of all, restores nature's balance.

CHAPTER 5 # Foot relaxation exercises and the thumb technique

To enable practical procedures to be understood and correctly followed, throughout this book certain views of the feet are referred to in a specific way.

VIEWS OF THE FEET

1 The plantar side of the foot represents the sole of the foot. *See Figure 5.1.*
2 The dorsal side is the front of the foot. *See Figure 5.2.*
3 The medial side represents the middle line of the foot, in line with your big toe. *See Figure 5.3.*
4 The lateral side is the outside edge of the foot, in line with the little toe. *See Figure 5.4.*

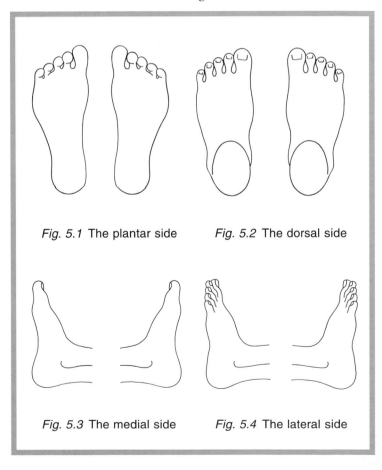

Fig. 5.1 The plantar side   *Fig. 5.2* The dorsal side

Fig. 5.3 The medial side   *Fig. 5.4* The lateral side

FOOT RELAXATION EXERCISES

Relaxation exercises are special techniques used at the beginning of a treatment, during a treatment and to end a treatment session.

They are used to enhance relaxation and to give the foot maximum movement. They can also be used if a specific system in the body creates extra sensitivities in the feet which may cause a little discomfort to the patient.

If we come across an extra sensitive point in the foot when working through a treatment session, we can follow on with the use of one or more relaxation exercises, this is very soothing to the patient.

The relaxation exercises are good for the student in training too, as they help them to become accustomed to handling feet and to maintaining contact with the patient through the treatment.

1 Side-to-side relaxation

Side-to-side relaxation

1 RIGHT FOOT

Figure 5.5 Commencing with the right foot and supporting the foot at the top, use a rocking, side-to-side movement – the foot should move quite swiftly.

2 LEFT FOOT

Figure 5.6 Exactly the same technique is employed when working on the left foot.

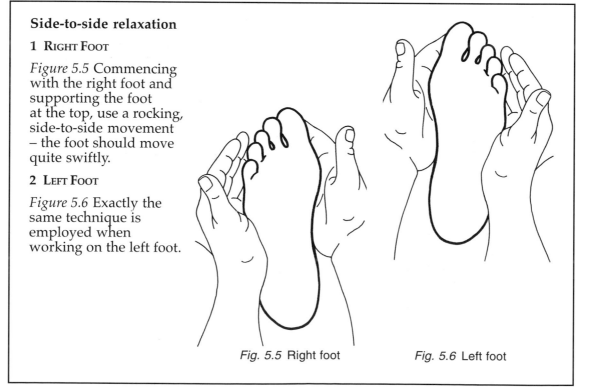

Fig. 5.5 Right foot   *Fig. 5.6* Left foot

2 Diaphragm relaxation

Diaphragm relaxation

1 RIGHT FOOT

Figure 5.7 Beginning with the right foot, place the right thumb on the commencement of the diaphragm line. As you move the thumb outwards towards the lateral side of the foot, bend the toes downwards on to your thumb. At no time should the thumb leave the surface of the foot.

When you have completed the exercise on the right foot, change over to the left foot.

2 LEFT FOOT

Figure 5.8 Now you will be supporting the left foot with the right hand and using the left thumb to commence. Change the direction when working on the left foot and place the left thumb on the lateral edge of the diaphragm line and work back to the medial side.

This is a great relaxant to the diaphragm muscle, and produces nice, slow, rhythmic breathing – almost putting the body into a 'sleeping mode' – and so is recommended as an exercise to start your treatment session.

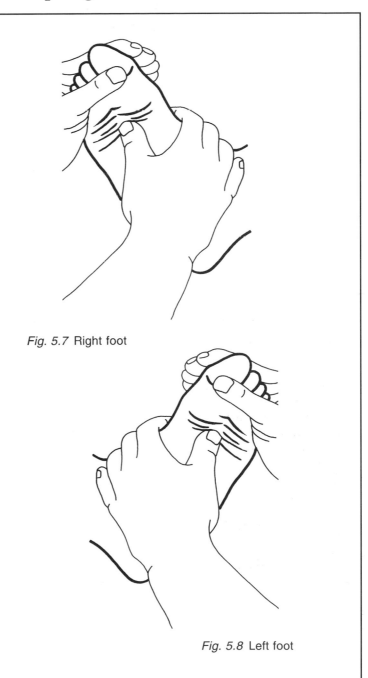

Fig. 5.7 Right foot

Fig. 5.8 Left foot

3 Metatarsal kneading

Metatarsal kneading

1 RIGHT FOOT

Figures 5.9 and 5.10
Commence with the right foot. Place the right fist on the plantar side of the right foot, and place the left hand over the dorsal side of the foot, using a pushing movement from the plantar side and a gentle squeezing movement from the dorsal side – this will create a kneading technique. This is a combined movement: both must be in harmony with each other.

2 LEFT FOOT

Figures 5.11 and 5.12
Work on the left foot. This time the left fist will be placed on the plantar side and the right hand on the dorsal.

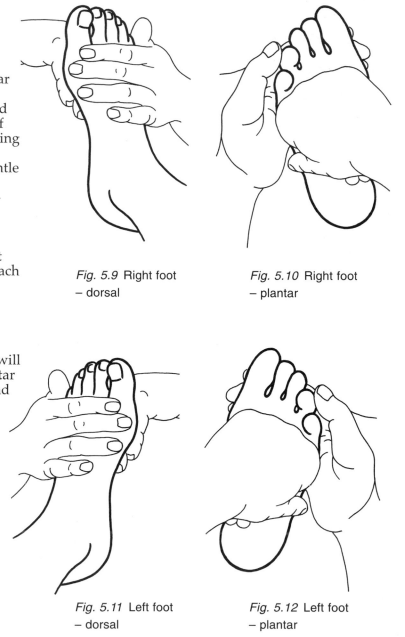

Fig. 5.9 Right foot – dorsal

Fig. 5.10 Right foot – plantar

Fig. 5.11 Left foot – dorsal

Fig. 5.12 Left foot – plantar

4 Ankle freeing

Ankle freeing

1 RIGHT FOOT

Figure 5.13 Commencing with the right foot, position the pads of the thumb joints in front of the ankle bones and rock the foot with a side-to-side motion.

2 LEFT FOOT

Figure 5.14 Repeat the same exercise on the left foot.

Ankle freeing is excellent for loosening up stiff ankles.

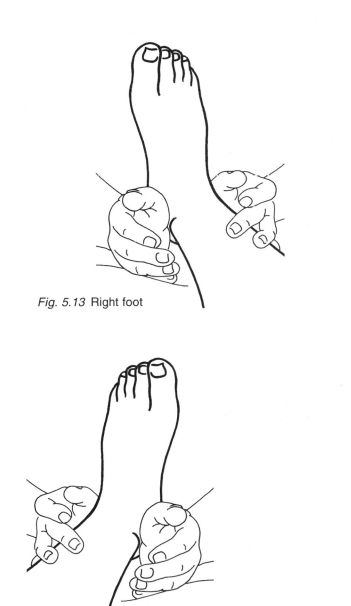

Fig. 5.13 Right foot

Fig. 5.14 Left foot

5 Undergrip

Undergrip

1 RIGHT FOOT

Figures 5.15 and 5.17
Place the left hand under the ankle (with thumb on lateral edge of the foot). Turn the foot in an inward direction, being sure to use a light, circling movement.

2 LEFT FOOT

Figures 5.16 and 5.18
Repeat the same exercise on the left foot, this time you must place the right hand under the ankle and then turn the foot inwards with the left hand.

A very relieving technique when treating those with swollen legs and ankles.

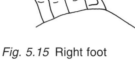

Fig. 5.15 Right foot

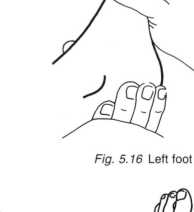

Fig. 5.16 Left foot

Direction of rotation

Figures 5.17 and 5.18 show the direction of rotation of the feet during the Undergrip relaxation exercise.

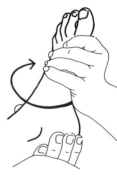

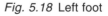

Fig. 5.17 Right foot

Fig. 5.18 Left foot

6 Overgrip

Overgrip

1 RIGHT FOOT

Figure 5.19 Place the left hand over the top of the right ankle, again making sure that the thumb of the left hand is on the lateral edge of the foot and use the same technique of rotation as in the Undergrip relaxation exercise.

2 LEFT FOOT

Figure 5.20 Reverse the above procedure placing the right hand over the top of the left ankle and rotate the foot as before.

This is another very relieving technique to use when treating those with swollen legs and ankles.

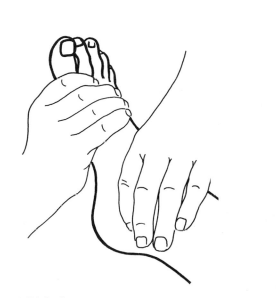

Fig. 5.19 Right foot

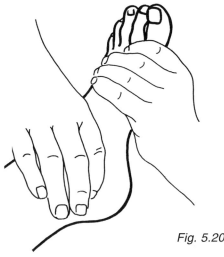

Fig. 5.20 Left foot

7 Foot moulding

Foot moulding

1 RIGHT FOOT

Figures 5.21 and 5.22
Support the right foot
– this time from the
lateral edge of the foot.
Gently sandwich the
foot between your two
hands and gently rotate
both hands. Both hands
must be in tune with
each other. The
movement resembles
the motions of the
wheels of a train.

2 LEFT FOOT

Figures 5.23 and 5.24
Move to the left foot
and repeat the same
technique.

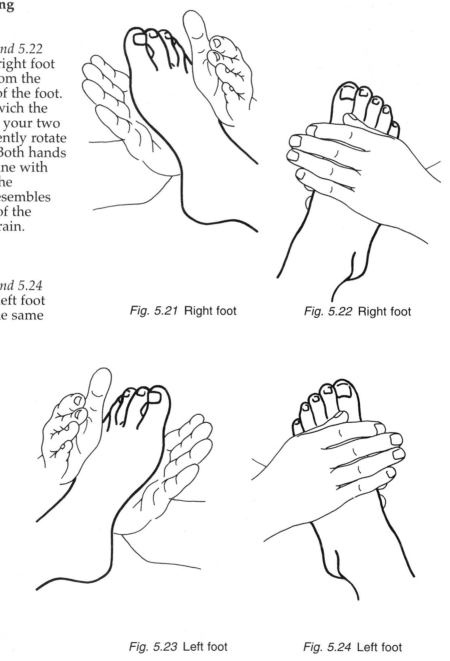

Fig. 5.21 Right foot

Fig. 5.22 Right foot

Fig. 5.23 Left foot

Fig. 5.24 Left foot

8 Rib cage relaxation

Rib cage relaxation

1 RIGHT FOOT

Figures 5.25 and *5.26* Apply pressure to the plantar side of the foot with your two thumbs. Use all the fingers of both hands and creep around the dorsal side of the foot.

2 LEFT FOOT

Figures 5.27 and *5.28* Repeat the above procedures on the left foot.

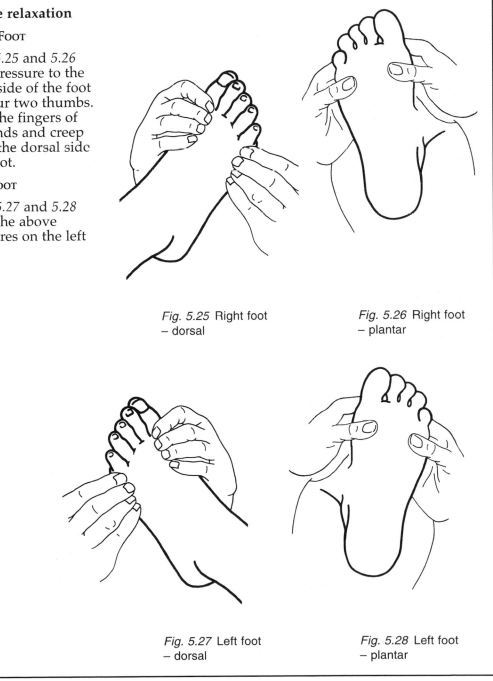

Fig. 5.25 Right foot
– dorsal

Fig. 5.26 Right foot
– plantar

Fig. 5.27 Left foot
– dorsal

Fig. 5.28 Left foot
– plantar

THE THUMB TECHNIQUE

The movement that we need to acquire with our thumb, in particular, is a forward creeping movement, bending from the first joint of the thumb. *See Figures 5.29, 5.30 and 5.31.*

We do not rotate in circles, hold a deep pressure for any length of time to any reflex point, or apply any oils or creams to the feet prior to a treatment session. An oily foot makes direct contact with the tiny reflex points in the feet impossible. It is quite in order to use a foot cream at the end of the treatment session.

We never use any wooden probes, electrical stimulating devices or anything of a similar nature. Why should we? Reflexology is a simple, effective science and is popular because of this simplicity. Nothing ever replaces the touch of the human hand.

The movement takes time to acquire because it is unusual for the thumb to work in this way. Acquiring sufficient pressure takes time, time to build up sufficient muscle power in your thumb and index finger. After all, your thumbs have never been called on to work in this way before.

The thumb technique
Visualise an old fashioned pin cushion with the pins distributed throughout at intervals of about 0.6 cm (a quarter of an inch). Bend your thumb and press the pin down into the pin cushion. Go to the next pin and do likewise. Combine tiny movements with a slow, deliberate movement travelling over the whole surface of the foot to make the whole treatment far more successful. We do not at any time work backwards, always on-going, forward creeping movements working towards the heart. *Figures 5.29, 5.30 and 5.31.*

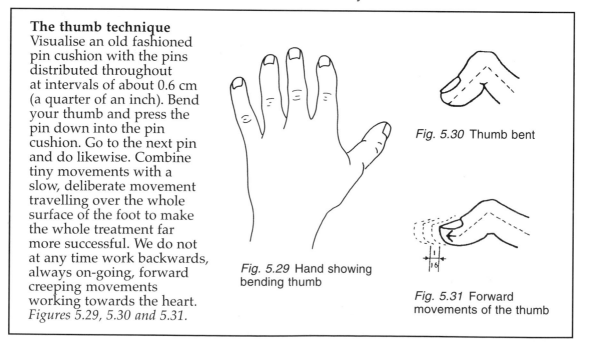

Fig. 5.29 Hand showing bending thumb

Fig. 5.30 Thumb bent

Fig. 5.31 Forward movements of the thumb

CHAPTER **6** The digestive system

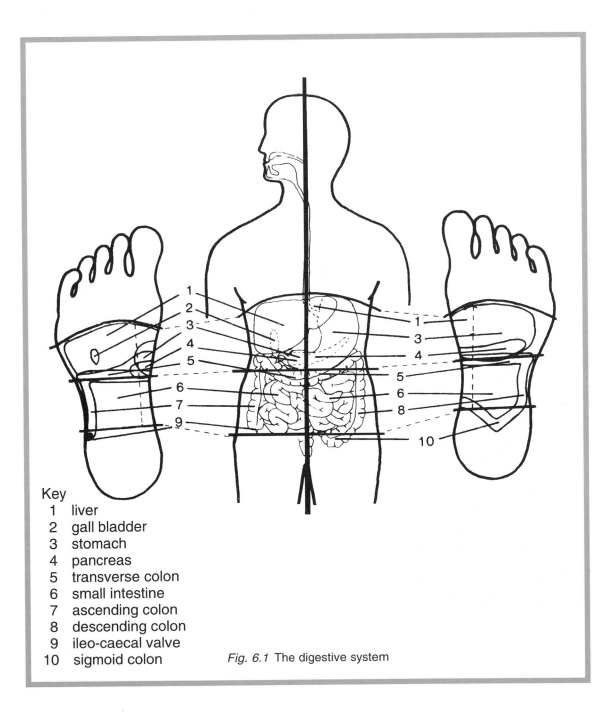

Key
1 liver
2 gall bladder
3 stomach
4 pancreas
5 transverse colon
6 small intestine
7 ascending colon
8 descending colon
9 ileo-caecal valve
10 sigmoid colon

Fig. 6.1 The digestive system

THE DIGESTIVE SYSTEM

See Figure 6.1. Digestion is the term used to describe the digestive processes which take place at different levels in the digestive system, also called the alimentary canal, to prepare food for absorption in the body.

The alimentary tract is a long tube through which food is digested and absorbed. The process begins at the mouth and terminates at the anus. The various organs have distinctive names although structurally they are remarkably similar. The main ones are the mouth, pharynx, oesophagus, stomach, liver, small intestine, large intestine, rectum and the anal canal.

Three types of accessory glands, namely, the salivary glands, liver and pancreas are not part of the digestive system but secrete digestive juices into it.

The complex digestive processes gradually simplify the food we eat until it is in a form suitable for absorption. All the energy the body needs comes from ingested food and drink.

More than any other system in the human body, the digestive system makes us aware when all is working efficiently and, equally, we are soon informed when the system is upset and in need of attention.

Hunger and the need to empty the bowels are two messages that we cannot ignore for long, as digestion is coordinated by the hypothalamus, hormones and nerves.

Indigestion causes the stomach to almost go into revolt and as rumblings and gurglings are felt and an unpleasant acid reflux action occurs, we really do feel completely out of sorts as our stomach either works overtime in an attempt to digest some extremely rich or spicy food which it is having difficulty in breaking down, or maybe we ate a meal very hurriedly, or perhaps we were worried and upset at the time.

The stomach is extremely sensitive to emotional upsets, so our mood and feelings affect the fine balance of the activity of this organ.

The increase in bowel disease, especially bowel cancer is linked to diet, the decrease in fibrous food since the introduction of the soft white bread loaf, a huge increase in the consumption of cakes, biscuits, and pies, and the increase of sugar in nearly everything that is packaged or in a jar, and we suffer from a constipated colon where waste food is kept in the body for far too long, a sure breeding ground for disease to manifest.

The entire digestive system relies on a strong muscular function to force our food through the digestive tract, this activity is called 'peristalsis'.

Whilst food is still in the mouth you have the choice to spit it out or swallow it. If it is swallowed, it then comes under the control of the autonomic nervous system where all the processes of digestion are not under your conscious control.

1 The mouth, pharynx and oesophagus

The mouth

See Figure 6.2. As soon as food enters the mouth it is chewed by our strong back teeth, our molars, and mixed with saliva which is produced by our salivary glands. As food is mixed with saliva, it becomes a soft mass, a bolus, and becomes easy to swallow.

We have three pairs of salivary glands: the parotid, submandibular and sublingual.

The pharynx

The pharynx carries food and air from the mouth towards the larynx and oesophagus. A flap of cartilage known as the epiglottis, folds over the entrance to the larynx as we swallow, thus preventing food entering the airway on its way to the oesophagus.

The oesophagus

Food is propelled along the oesophagus by muscular force into the stomach.

At the lower end of the oesophagus is a strong circular muscle called the cardiac sphincter muscle which guards the entrance to the stomach, preventing the highly acid gastric juice from splashing up into the oesophagus.

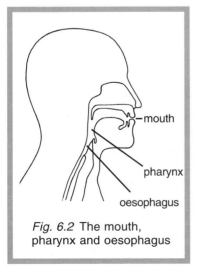

Fig. 6.2 The mouth, pharynx and oesophagus

2 The liver and gall bladder

See Figure 6.3. The liver and gall bladder, as well as the pancreas, are closely connected with the digestive tract but are not actually part of it.

The liver

The liver lies on the right hand side of the body and is one of the most important organs in the human body. It is wedge shaped, very vascular and has some amazing chemical processing abilities. It has two lobes, the left lobe being smaller than the right, and tiny tubes and billions of cells form the internal structure of the liver.

The liver is a great detoxifier. It produces bile, cholesterol and vitamin B12 and stores vitamins A, D, E and K as well as iron, copper and some water soluble vitamins such as folic acid, vitamin B, pyridoxine and niacin.

The liver converts glucose to glucogen, and it converts stored fat into a form which can be used by the body to provide energy and heat. The liver deals efficiently with the detoxification of drugs and toxins and the ethanol which is found in alcohol.

The bile produced by the liver is vital to digestion, emulsifying fats and also providing lubrication for the bowel.

Bile consists of water, bile pigment and bile salts, cholesterol, mineral salts, and mucus. Up to 1,000 ml of bile is secreted by the liver daily.

The gall bladder

The gall bladder is a pear shaped sac which lies under the liver.

The cystic artery supplies blood to the gall bladder, which has a muscular layer within its wall. The gall bladder stores the bile and as the muscular wall contracts, bile passes through the bile ducts to the duodenum which is the first part of the small intestine.

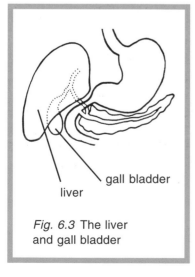

gall bladder
liver

Fig. 6.3 The liver and gall bladder

3 The stomach, pancreas and the Islets of Langerhans

The stomach

See Figure 6.4. The stomach is a hollow elastic 'C' shaped sac with strong muscular contracting functions. The fundus or top of the stomach is situated just underneath our heart and the base joins the first part of the small intestine called the duodenum. A strong muscular ring called the pyloric sphincter lies at the base of the stomach and relaxes and contracts as food leaves the stomach and enters the small intestine.

The stomach wall is composed of four main layers.
i) The mucosa is the lining of the stomach.
ii) The submucosa, a layer of connective tissue lies beneath the mucosa.
iii) The third layer consists of longitudinal, circular and oblique layers of muscle and waves of peristaltic action move food through the entire digestive tract.
iv) The serosa is the outer coat.

Gastric glands in the wall of the stomach secrete hydrochloric acid and enzymes. The hydrochloric acid kills bacteria and breaks down the connective tissues in meat.

The main enzyme secreted in the the gastric juice is pepsin which starts protein digestion. Small amounts of water, salts and alcohol are absorbed through the mucosa of the stomach.

The intrinsic factor, which is a protein, is necessary for the absorption of vitamin B.

The flow of gastric juices before food reaches the stomach is due to the stimulation of the vagus nerve which is activated by the sight, smell or taste of food.

The length of time that the stomach takes to digest its contents depends on the type of food eaten. A fatty meal remains in the stomach the longest.

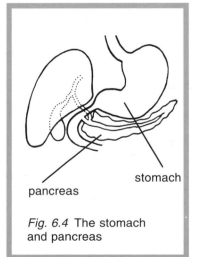

stomach

pancreas

Fig. 6.4 The stomach and pancreas

The pancreas

See Figure 6.5. The pancreas is a pale grey gland about 12 to 15 cm long which is situated near the epigastric region of the abdominal cavity. It consists of a broad head, a body and a narrow tail.

The head lies in the curve of the duodenum; the body lies behind the stomach and the tail is in front of the left kidney and just reaches the spleen. The abdominal aorta and the inferior vena cava lie behind the gland.

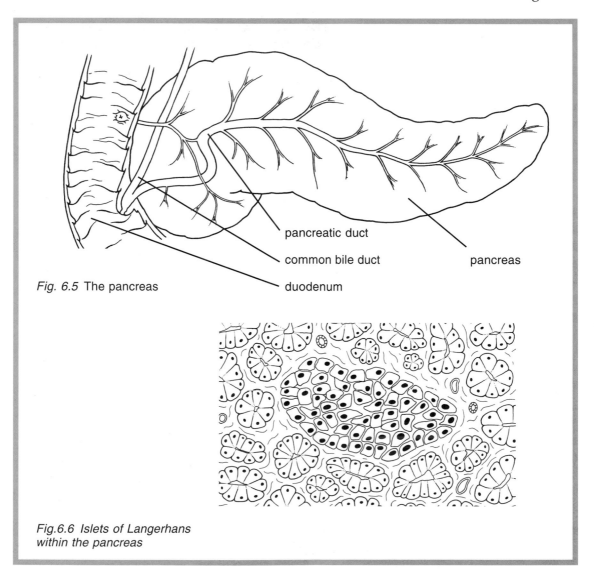

pancreatic duct

common bile duct   pancreas

Fig. 6.5 The pancreas   duodenum

Fig.6.6 Islets of Langerhans within the pancreas

The Islets of Langerhans

See Figure 6.6. The Islets of Langerhans are the endocrine areas of the pancreas. The alpha cells secrete glucagon and the beta cells produce insulin. These hormones work in opposition to control the glucose blood sugar level. Inadequate production of insulin results in the disease diabetes mellitus.

The remainder of the pancreas produces pancreatic juice containing enzymes secreted in an alkaline juice which are released into the duodenum via the pancreatic duct to help in the digestive process of carbohydrates, proteins and fats.

4 The small and large intestine, rectum and anal canal

The small intestine

See Figure 6.7. The small intestine is really a continuation of the stomach, the first part of the small intestine being the duodenum which is about 25 cm long and encircles the head of the pancreas.

The jejunum is the middle part of the small intestine and is about 2 metres long.

The ileum is about 3 metres in length and ends at the ileo-caecal valve which joins the small and large intestine. This little valve prevents backflow of waste material once it has left the small intestine.

The large intestine

The large intestine has strong muscular movements which propel waste matter along the colon towards the rectum, this muscular action is known as peristalsis and is active throughout the entire digestive system.

The large intestine is about 1.5 metres long, beginning at the caecum and terminating at the rectum and anal canal, deep in the pelvis. The space it encloses is larger than that of the small intestine. It forms an arch around the small intestine. The large intestine is divided into the caecum, ascending colon, transverse colon, descending colon, sigmoid or pelvic colon, rectum and anal canal.

The ascending colon passes up from the caecum to the level of the liver where it bends acutely to the left at the hepatic flexure to become the transverse colon.

The transverse colon is a loop of colon which extends across the abdominal cavity to the front of the jejunum and the stomach to the area of the spleen where it forms the splenic flexure by bending acutely downwards to become the descending colon.

The descending colon passes down the left side of the abdominal cavity, then curves towards the mid line. After it enters the true pelvis, it is known as the pelvic colon.

The pelvic colon or sigmoid is an S-shaped curve in the pelvis which continues downwards to become the rectum.

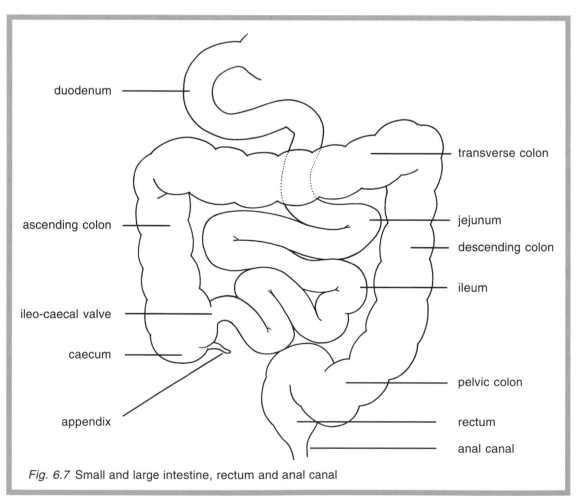

Fig. 6.7 Small and large intestine, rectum and anal canal

The rectum

The rectum is a slightly dilated part of the colon which is about 13 cm long. It leads from the pelvic colon (sigmoid) and terminates in the anal canal.

The anal canal

The anal canal is a short canal about 3.8 cm long in the adult and leads from the rectum to the exterior. There are two sphincter muscles which control the anus. The internal sphincter consisting of smooth muscle fibres is under the control of the autonomic nervous system and the external sphincter formed by striated muscle, is under voluntary control.

Faecal matter moves through the large intestine at a slow speed permitting the reabsorption of approximately 1.3 litres (2.5 pt) of water every day.

Food absorption and elimination of waste

The lining of the small intestine has millions of projections called villi. The villi increase the surface area of the small intestine for digestion and absorption of nutrients.

Secretion of digestive juices is stimulated by hormones and by stretching due to contents. The intestinal glands are stimulated to release their fluid mainly by local reflexes that occur when the small intestine is stretched.

Therefore the small intestine absorbs all the necessary nutrients from our food, secretes the intestinal fluid, completes the chemical digestion of carbohydrates, protein and fats, and protects against the invasion of infection.

The mucosa of the large intestine lacks villi and produces no digestive enzymes.

The functions of the large intestine are absorption of sodium and water, incubation of bacteria which produce vitamin K and some of the B complex vitamins, and elimination of wastes in the form of undigested and unabsorbed food and bile pigments.

The longer waste material is left in the bowel, the more likelihood there is of diseases occurring in the colon. A famous medical herbal college believes that 'Death Begins in the Colon'!

Due to the western way of living over the last 30 years or so, bowel disorders and diseases are on the increase, particularly bowel cancer.

Constipation too is very common in those whose diets are very low in fibre. Stress and lack of exercise also have a disastrous effect on the colon.

CHAPTER 7 Practical procedures for working the digestive system

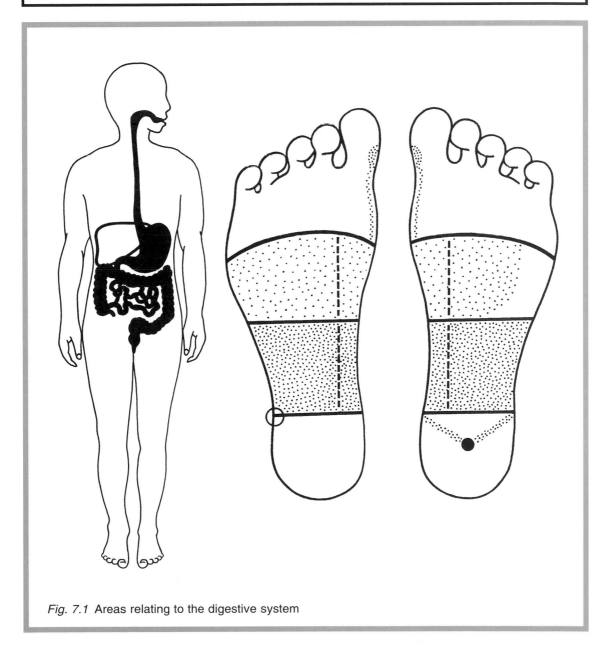

Fig. 7.1 Areas relating to the digestive system

1 The liver area – *right foot* Zones 1 2 3 4 5 (and Zone 1 on left foot)

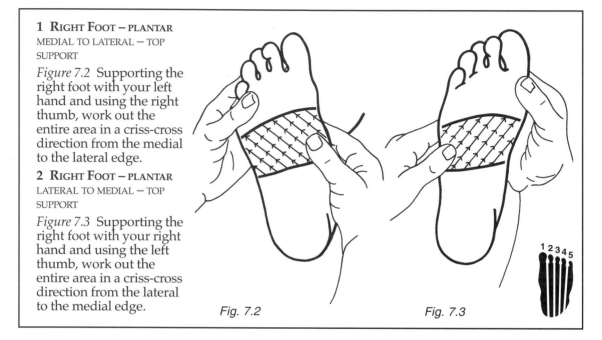

1 RIGHT FOOT – PLANTAR
MEDIAL TO LATERAL – TOP
SUPPORT

Figure 7.2 Supporting the
right foot with your left
hand and using the right
thumb, work out the
entire area in a criss-cross
direction from the medial
to the lateral edge.

2 RIGHT FOOT – PLANTAR
LATERAL TO MEDIAL – TOP
SUPPORT

Figure 7.3 Supporting the
right foot with your right
hand and using the left
thumb, work out the
entire area in a criss-cross
direction from the lateral
to the medial edge.

Fig. 7.2   Fig. 7.3

2 The stomach and pancreas areas – *left foot* Zones 1 2 3 4

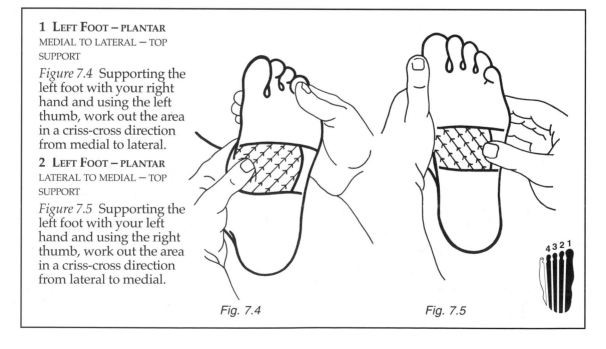

1 LEFT FOOT – PLANTAR
MEDIAL TO LATERAL – TOP
SUPPORT

Figure 7.4 Supporting the
left foot with your right
hand and using the left
thumb, work out the area
in a criss-cross direction
from medial to lateral.

2 LEFT FOOT – PLANTAR
LATERAL TO MEDIAL – TOP
SUPPORT

Figure 7.5 Supporting the
left foot with your left
hand and using the right
thumb, work out the area
in a criss-cross direction
from lateral to medial.

Fig. 7.4   Fig. 7.5

3 The ileo-caecal valve – *right foot* Zone 5

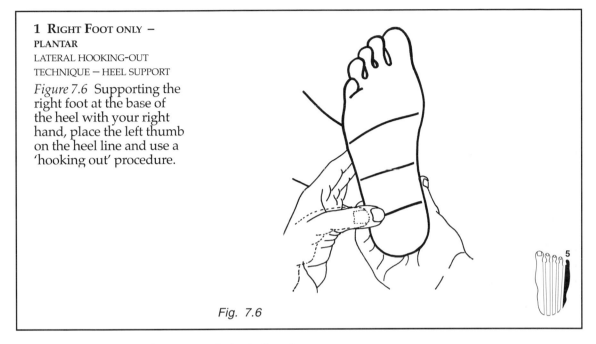

1 RIGHT FOOT ONLY –
PLANTAR
LATERAL HOOKING-OUT
TECHNIQUE – HEEL SUPPORT

Figure 7.6 Supporting the right foot at the base of the heel with your right hand, place the left thumb on the heel line and use a 'hooking out' procedure.

Fig. 7.6

4 The intestinal area – *(a) right foot* Zones 1 2 3 4 5

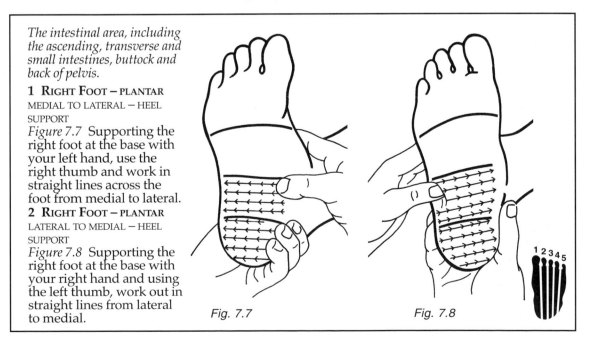

The intestinal area, including the ascending, transverse and small intestines, buttock and back of pelvis.

1 RIGHT FOOT – PLANTAR
MEDIAL TO LATERAL – HEEL
SUPPORT
Figure 7.7 Supporting the right foot at the base with your left hand, use the right thumb and work in straight lines across the foot from medial to lateral.

2 RIGHT FOOT – PLANTAR
LATERAL TO MEDIAL – HEEL
SUPPORT
Figure 7.8 Supporting the right foot at the base with your right hand and using the left thumb, work out in straight lines from lateral to medial.

Fig. 7.7   Fig. 7.8

5 The intestinal area – *(b) left foot* Zones 1 2 3 4 5

Transverse, descending and small intestines, including the buttock and back of the pelvis which are situated below the heel line.

1 LEFT FOOT – PLANTAR
MEDIAL TO LATERAL – HEEL SUPPORT
Figure 7.9 Supporting the left foot in your right hand at the base and using the left thumb, work out in straight lines from medial to lateral.

2 LEFT FOOT – PLANTAR
LATERAL TO MEDIAL – HEEL SUPPORT
Figure 7.10 Supporting the left foot at the base with your left hand and using your right thumb, work across in straight lines from lateral to medial.

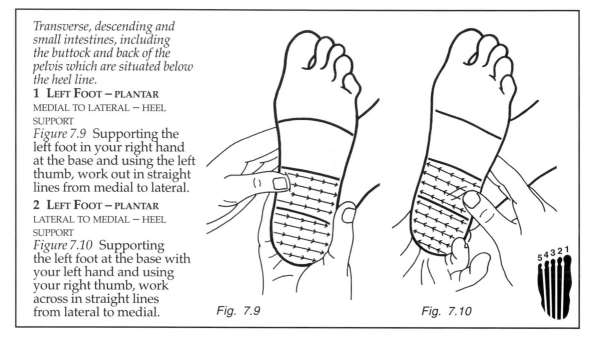

Fig. 7.9   Fig. 7.10

6 The sigmoid or pelvic colon – *left foot* Zone 3

Area representing the sigmoid or pelvic colon, the bend, left foot.

1 LEFT FOOT – PLANTAR
MID TO MEDIAL – HEEL SUPPORT
Figure 7.11 Supporting the left foot at the base with your left hand, place the right thumb on the mid point and work towards the medial edge.

2 LEFT FOOT – PLANTAR
MID TO LATERAL – HEEL SUPPORT
Figure 7.11 Change direction and support the foot at the base with your right hand and work with the left thumb towards the lateral edge.

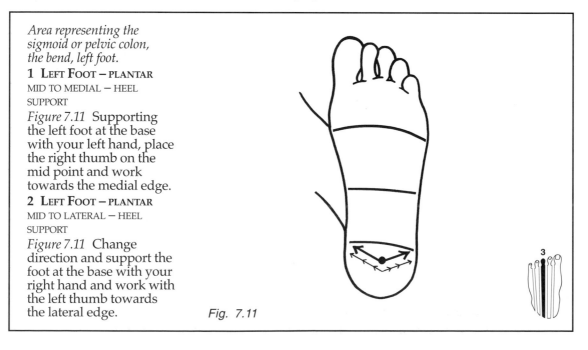

Fig. 7.11

CHAPTER 8 The respiratory system

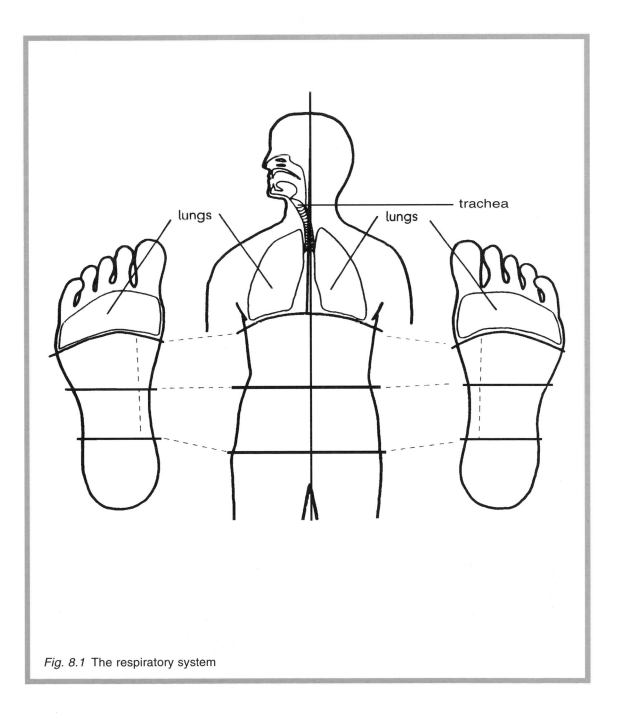

Fig. 8.1 The respiratory system

THE RESPIRATORY SYSTEM

The function of our lungs and heart provides the body with oxygenated blood, which is necessary for the survival of every single cell. Each lung expands and contracts between 15 and 80 times a minute, not only to supply the body with oxygen but to expel the waste gas – carbon dioxide.

The body is unable to store oxygen so we need to breathe continuously for survival. Our respiratory rate drops to a slow rate during sleep and can increase dramatically if we are running for our life or climbing a mountain when huge effort is needed, not only by the respiratory system and the circulation but by the entire human form.

Respiration (breathing) supplies the cells of the body with oxygen and removes carbon dioxide and includes gas exchange between lungs and blood, transport of gases through the body by the blood, gas exchange between blood and cells, and cellular respiration (use of oxygen by the cells and production of carbon dioxide by the cells).

The respiratory system comprises nose, pharynx, larynx, trachea, bronchi, bronchioles, two lungs, which are spongy bags, pulmonary vessels, and the dependency of the large diaphragmatic muscle, which acts as a bellows to the lungs. The intercostal muscles between each rib allow the expansion of the thoracic cavity. When we take in a deep breath our diaphragm muscle descends and the rib cage expands: this is how we obtain oxygen in our lungs. *See Figures 8.2 and 8.3.*

We normally breathe in and out about 10 to 17 times each minute but in the case of a respiratory condition this can increase alarmingly as the congested airways reduce the overall oxygen capacity.

The respiratory system involves air going into and coming out of the lungs. As we breathe through our nose tiny hairs prevent particles from entering the nasal cavities behind. The nasal passages also warm up or cool down air, creating a pleasant humidifying state in our respiratory system. Ciliated mucous membrane which lines the respiratory system also traps particles of dust and other irritants. The smallest bronchioles and the alveoli are not equipped with cells with cilia or with mucus.

If you are a mouth breather you will be subjected to more sore throats than usual and will probably snore during sleep.

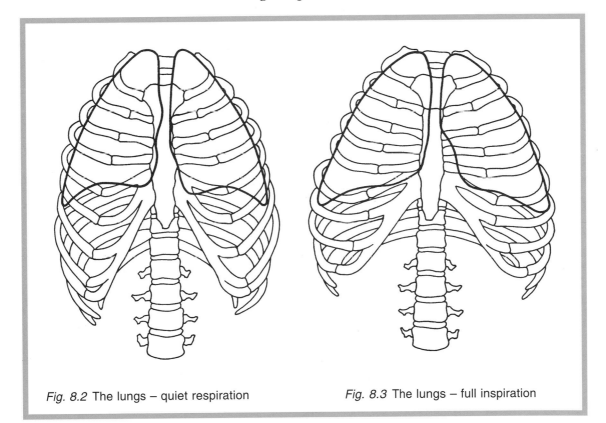

Fig. 8.2 The lungs – quiet respiration   *Fig. 8.3* The lungs – full inspiration

1 The lungs

Each lung is cone-shaped with a slightly concave base that sits on the diaphragm. The lungs are protected by the rib cage which is quite flexible having intercostal muscles between each rib space, together they form one of the largest organs in the body.

A membrane surrounds each lung, this is called the pleural membrane, and is filled with pleural fluid. This prevents friction building up as the lungs expand and recoil.

2 The trachea, bronchial tubes and bronchioles

The trachea

Air breathed in through the nose or through the mouth becomes warm and moist on passing through the nasal passages, pharynx and larynx (voice box). During swallowing a flap of tissue, the epiglottis, automatically closes off the larynx so food cannot enter the lower airway. Air continues down to the trachea.

Bronchial tubes

Air passes from the trachea through two bronchi to the lungs. The intricate network of air passages that supply the lungs resembles an inverted tree with the trachea being the trunk. Branches extend outwards and are called bronchial tubes and bronchioles.

Bronchioles

Inside the lungs, bronchi branch out into small tubes called bronchioles. There are about 30,000 bronchioles in each lung. Bronchioles end in alveolar sacs – clusters of tiny chambers known as alveoli. *See Figure 8.4.*

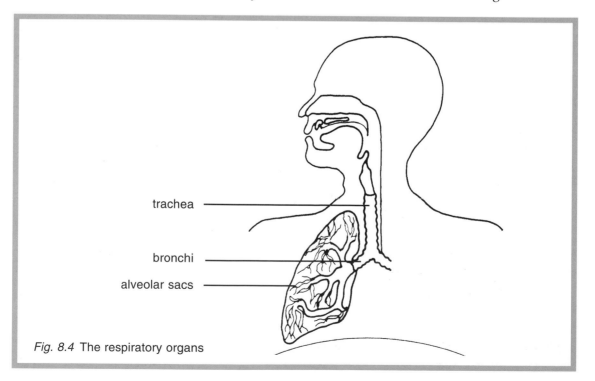

trachea

bronchi

alveolar sacs

Fig. 8.4 The respiratory organs

3 Alveoli

The air sacs in the lungs are called alveoli, and they are expandable, thin-walled structures through which the exchange of oxygen and carbon dioxide takes place. Their thin walls support a network of capillaries, the tiny tubes containing blood. Air is inhaled and oxygen diffuses from the alveoli into the blood and is transported to body cells. Carbon dioxide from cells is conveyed in blood to the lungs. It diffuses from the pulmonary capillaries into the alveoli and is then exhaled. Spread flat, the alveoli in a pair of lungs would cover half a tennis court.

White blood cells are present on the surface of each alveoli, which resemble bunches of small seedless grapes. The white blood cells ingest and destroy airborne irritants, such as bacteria and grass pollen.

If disease invades the lung causing destruction of these minute alveoli there is less surface area for gaseous exchange and breathlessness occurs, which ultimately places a stress on the heart. *See Figure 8.5.*

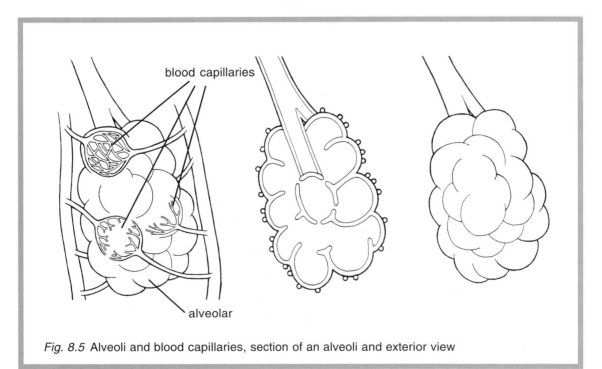

blood capillaries

alveolar

Fig. 8.5 Alveoli and blood capillaries, section of an alveoli and exterior view

4 The larynx

Sounds are created through special structures in the body's airway. Exhaled air flows through the larynx or the voice box, a broad part of the upper windpipe protected by tough cartilage that forms the Adam's apple. Two bands of tissue called 'vocal cords' form a V shaped opening across the larynx. As we speak these tighten, narrowing the opening. Exhaled air vibrates the cords and produces sounds; the longer the cords, the higher the pitch. Sounds carry with different positions of the tongue, lips and teeth. The nasal cavities give resonance to the voice.

Respiratory conditions benefiting from reflexology

The types of conditions that the reflexologist will be able to relieve and assist are bronchitis, asthma, emphysema, and all the other respiratory tract infections which will be covered in Chapter 9: Practical Procedures for Working the Respiratory System.

Poor functioning in the respiratory system often has its root cause in digestion and it may be difficult for you to accept that, in order to get good relief from a respiratory condition, the digestive system needs to be worked – but that is so very true.

There is evidence to show when some infants are fed with cows milk and wheat based products at a young age, an allergic reaction can start up in the mucous membranes of the body, and remember we have this membrane lining the entire digestive system as well as the respiratory system.

Those most likely to suffer from allergies are babies with a family history of allergic reactive illnesses, i.e. migraine, (80 per cent of migraine is caused by an allergy), hay fever, eczema, hives, or other irritating rashes. Some babies are born with eczema which has been caused by a certain food or foods that the mother has been eating, maybe in excess, for as we all know many pregnant mothers have certain strange cravings for all manner of foods, and often the food we crave is the very one that we are allergic to.

Those who suffer from allergies have a more delicate constitution than others who can eat exactly what they like at any time without any adverse reaction from the body at all. I usually try to compare the individual constitutions of people as some of us who have a constitution of a 'Mini' and another a 'Rolls Royce' and we all know that you can get far more performance from the latter.

Babies, who after all were born without teeth, were really meant to have nothing more than breast milk until they had grinding teeth, but these do not appear until the end of the second year. If we, therefore, respected the laws of nature we would realise that the infant was not meant to take any solid food into his body until the end of the second year. At that time the digestive system would have matured and allergic reactions would be far less likely.

The ingestion of various foods at a very young age sets up an inflammatory state in the body and also puts a stress on the kidney function. Your child may start suffering from ear infections, a constant running nose, sore throats, or maybe an outbreak of eczema.

This is Mother Nature desperately trying to give her silent signals that all is not well in the child's body. We are all exactly what we eat and any catarrhal or infected state in a baby has to be due to food that is not suitable.

Breast feeding is always the best, the quality of milk as well as the quantity changes with the demands of the baby: as the child gets older and needs a higher fat content in his food, nature adjusts this need.

Breast fed babies do not suffer from constipation, so a good eliminating process of waste products is also guaranteed. You do not get this when feeding with powdered formulaes.

When a young baby is suffering from an acute ear infection, the mother will of course go to the doctor for help, earache is very painful and debilitating. The doctor will undoubtedly treat the infection by prescribing an antibiotic. Antibiotics have quite a disastrous effect on the digestive system as they destroy the flora, the friendly bacteria which keeps the intestinal tract healthy. Here we start a never ending circle of problems, more ear infections, more antibiotics, and more damage to the very area that was in a sensitive state to start with.

There is no way that you can suppress nature. If you suppress the ear, nose and throat with constant antibiotics, nature will direct her way of eliminating the problem to another exit, and the progress of illness is usually the removal of the tonsils and adenoids in an attempt to alleviate the constant infections.

Tonsils and adenoids are lymphatic glands, the first line of defence in the body. They may well help the ear nose or throat infections, but the infection will then have a very easy direct access down to the lungs. No adenoids or tonsils in the way to absorb the bacteria, so the next port of call will be the lungs!

It is probable that the child will have attacks of what doctors refer to as wheezy bronchitis. The treatment will be yet more prescriptions for antibiotics, and if these do not help immediately then various bronchial inhalers are used to help expand the inflamed and infected bronchial tubes.

The bronchial dilating drugs work by affecting the nerve signals that control the contraction and relaxation of the bronchiole muscles. This relaxation ultimately gives more space for the air to come in and out of the lungs. Corticosteroid drugs, usually inhaled, widen the bronchial tubes thus lessening the inflammation.

However, all asthmatic drugs are not without their side effects and they can make the child tense and wound up, simply because they put the body into a 'flee or fight' state. The child may have behavioural problems, difficulty in sleeping or become aggressive, which is totally out of character from the norm.

Tension triggers an asthmatic attack, so here we have the progression of disease caused by poor management from a very young age.

Vaccinations also play their part and it is well known by those who work in the complementary field of medicine or naturopaths, that the huge increase in asthma is due to the whooping cough vaccine.

Yes, you may say, but what about the risk of death through whooping cough? There are many deaths caused as the result of asthma, and the tendency to the over-use of drugs to ease attacks. These we do not hear about!

If you took your young baby to a naturopath, or herbalist he would concentrate his efforts on helping the digestive system, by giving either homocopathic or herbal preparations. Great attention would be given to the child's diet – the removal of all dairy and wheat products, the use of goats milk or soya in replacement for powdered formulaes, and only vegetables, rices and some pureed fruits.

This basic, bland diet would be followed for many months until the large grinding teeth appear, which is a signal from Mother Nature that the digestive system is now mature and can start taking a variety of different foods.

The removal of dairy and wheat products would give the inflammation and congestion in the digestive system a time to heal and allergic reaction to food would be far less likely.

In industrialised countries, respiratory disorders are very common. The huge increase in road and air traffic pollutes our atmosphere and this plus the use of chemical sprays in farming give us a toxic, polluted environment. Our fruit and vegetables not only grow in chemically treated soil, but are sprayed with strong insecticides in order to give the housewife that perfect fruit and vegetable without a blemish.

We are therefore ingesting chemicals as well as inhaling them from the environment. By the use of peak flow meters, doctors are now able to measure the volume of air in the lungs. This method of volume testing is used extensively when treating asthmatic children.

Despite the government health warnings on cigarettes and the knowledge that cigarette smoking is the main cause of lung cancer, and that if smoking was abolished 89 per cent of lung cancer would disappear, the remaining 11 per cent of sufferers would be those who have been subjected to passive smoking or who are working in flour mills, or with asbestos.

Lung cancer was predominantly a male disease, but since women have become heavy smokers, the incident of cancer is steadily rising. It is the tar content in tobacco that causes the cancer along with a mixture of hundreds of different chemicals. The nicotine causes the addiction.

Silicosis is the world's most common occupational lung disease, caused by silica dust: coal miners and stone masons are particularly at risk. Lung tissue of chronic smokers and of those who work in dirty industries contains large, blackened areas where carbon particles have been deposited. This tissue does not expand and severely restricts the functioning of the lungs.

Asthma is increasing in to-day's society, and has doubled in the past two decades. There are various reasons for this, as I have discussed: diet is a big factor, pollution of our atmosphere another, and western 'stress' a third.

CHAPTER 9 Practical procedures for working the respiratory system

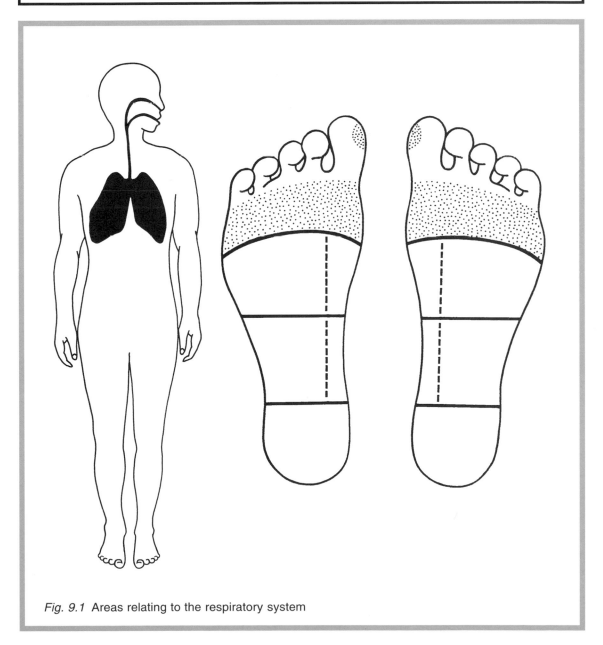

Fig. 9.1 Areas relating to the respiratory system

1 The lung area – (a) right foot Zones 1 2 3 4 5

1 RIGHT FOOT – PLANTAR
MEDIAL TO LATERAL – TOP
SUPPORT

Figure 9.2 Supporting the right foot with your left hand at the top and using the right thumb work up the foot in straight lines from medial to lateral.

2 RIGHT FOOT – PLANTAR
LATERAL TO MEDIAL – TOP
SUPPORT

Figure 9.3 Supporting the right foot with your right hand at the top and using the left thumb work up the foot in straight lines from lateral to medial.

Separate each toe as you proceed.

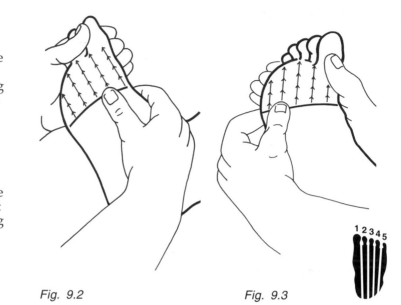

Fig. 9.2   Fig. 9.3

2 The lung/breast area – (b) right foot Zones 1 2 3 4 5

1 RIGHT FOOT – DORSAL
MEDIAL TO LATERAL – TOP
SUPPORT

Figure 9.4 Supporting the right foot with your left fist and using the right index finger proceed downwards from medial to lateral.

2 RIGHT FOOT – DORSAL
LATERAL TO MEDIAL – TOP
SUPPORT

Figure 9.5 Supporting the right foot with your right fist and using the left index finger proceed downwards from lateral to medial.

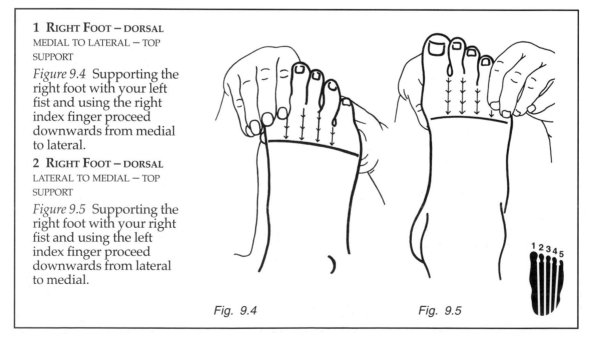

Fig. 9.4   Fig. 9.5

3 The lung area – (a) left foot Zones 1 2 3 4 5

1 LEFT FOOT – PLANTAR
MEDIAL TO LATERAL – TOP
SUPPORT

Figure 9.6 Supporting the left foot with the right hand and using the left thumb work up the foot in straight lines from medial to lateral.

2 LEFT FOOT – PLANTAR
LATERAL TO MEDIAL – TOP
SUPPORT

Figure 9.7 Supporting the left foot with the left hand and using the right thumb work up the foot in straight lines from lateral to medial.

Separate each toe as you proceed.

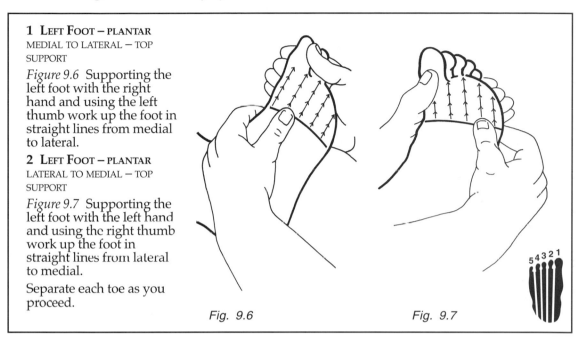

Fig. 9.6   Fig. 9.7

4 The lung/breast area – (b) left foot Zones 1 2 3 4 5

1 LEFT FOOT – DORSAL
MEDIAL TO LATERAL – TOP
SUPPORT

Figure 9.8 Supporting the left foot with your right fist and using the left index finger proceed downwards from medial to lateral.

2 LEFT FOOT – DORSAL
LATERAL TO MEDIAL – TOP
SUPPORT

Figure 9.9 Supporting the left foot with your left fist and using the right index finger proceed downwards from lateral to medial.

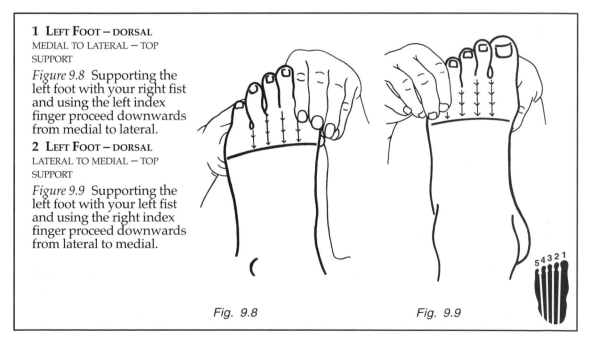

Fig. 9.8   Fig. 9.9

Position of the lungs within the thorax. The ribcage protects the lungs and vital organs.

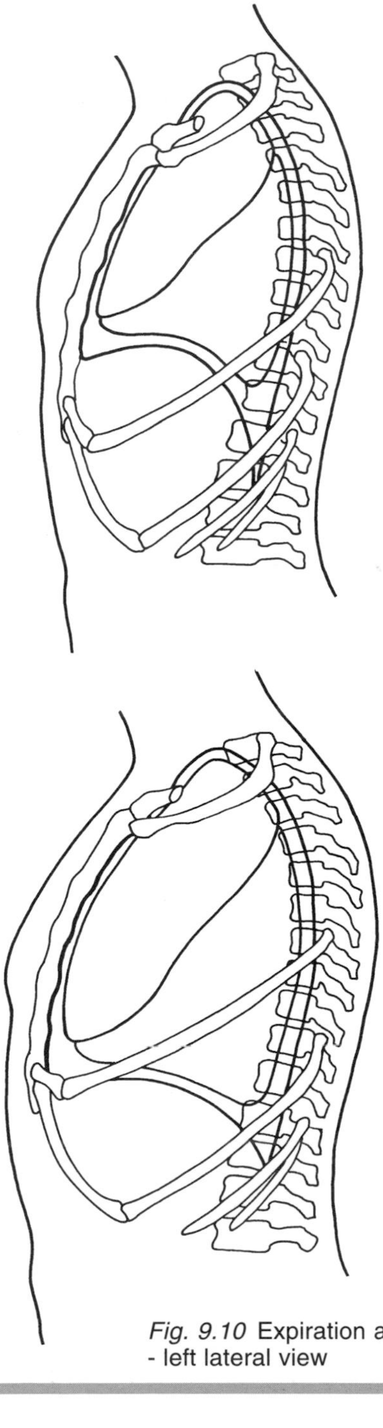

Fig. 9.10 Expiration and inspiration
- left lateral view

CHAPTER 10 The circulatory system

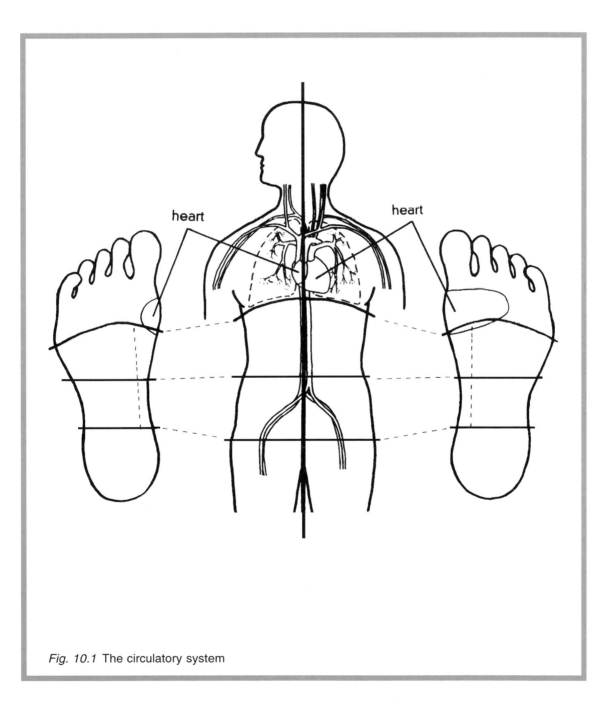

Fig. 10.1 The circulatory system

THE CIRCULATORY SYSTEM

As a dynamic pump, the heart is an amazingly sophisticated piece of equipment for supplying the body with energy. Indeed, its mechanics are so efficient that they are easily taken for granted.

The heart starts its life as two beating tubes which are able to be picked up on sophisticated monitoring equipment on the 16th day after conception. The heart has the responsibility to force oxygenated blood around the body through a network of blood vessels: arteries, veins and capillaries that would circle the earth two and a half times.

The heart is a cone-shaped, hollow organ, about the size of its owner's fist and lies in the thoracic cavity between the lungs – a little more to the left than the right. *See Figure 10.2.* The apex is about 9 cm to the left of the midline, i.e. a little below the nipple. The base extends to the level of the 2nd rib. The left lung overlaps the left side of the heart, the heart and lungs being protected and enclosed by the rib cage.

The wall of the heart consists of three layers. From the inside out, the layers are the endocardium (the smooth lining), the myocardium (heart muscle) and pericardium (strong sac for the heart).

The heart is a double pump. The right and left sides are completely separated by a wall or septum. The heart has four chambers. The upper two chambers of the heart are the atria and the lower two chambers are the ventricles.

Valves are situated between the ventricles and atria and open and close according to the changes of pressure in the chambers. The valve between the right atrium and the right ventricle is the tricuspid valve. The valve on the left side is the bicuspid valve. When the pressure in the atria is greater than that in the ventricles, they open. Valves guard the exits from the ventricles. Between the left ventricle and the aorta is the aortic valve, and the one between the right ventricle and the pulmonary artery is the pulmonary valve. The valves only allow the blood to flow in one direction.

The membranous bag that surrounds the heart, the

pericardium, has two layers: the outer layer which is called the parietal membrane and the visceral membrane is the inner layer.

In normal circulation both parts of the heart pump out the same amount of blood after each beat and take in the same amount as they pump out. The control of the speed at which the heart beats is organised by the vagus nerve, the resting rate is usually about 70 beats per minute. During exercise or stress the heart rate increases dramatically.

The main muscular beat is controlled by the myocardium – from the Greek muos: muscle and kardia: heart. This specialised type of muscle can work tirelessly for three score years and ten and often much longer without (a) breaking down, (b) needing replacement parts and (c) needing replacing altogether.

No other pump has ever or could ever be produced by man that could work so tirelessly, efficiently and silently as the human heart.

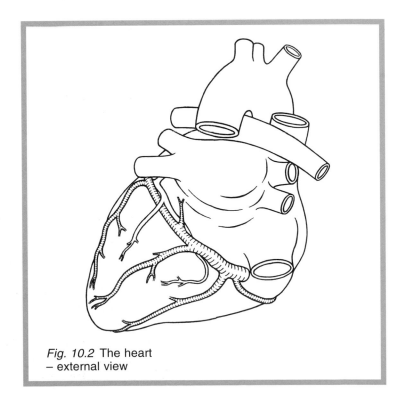

Fig. 10.2 The heart
– external view

1 Arteries, veins, capillaries and red blood cells

Our blood is carried through a complicated network of arteries, veins and capillaries. Arteries have much thicker walls than veins and capillaries as they carry blood at force, expanding to absorb the surge of blood and then contracting until the next heart beat.

Arteries

Arteries carry blood at high pressure so if an artery is cut open blood will spurt out at high pressure, while a slow steady flow of blood escapes from a vein. Arteries do not have valves.

Veins

Deoxygenated blood returning to the heart through the veins is at low pressure: its movement is helped by a succession of one-way valves that prevent backflow. Valves are in their abundance in the veins of the lower limbs where blood must flow a considerable distance against the force of gravity, when the individual is standing or lying down.

Capillaries

The smallest arterioles (arteries) break up into a number of minute vessels called capillaries. The walls of capillaries consist of just one single layer so are very fragile. Capillaries form a vast network which link the smallest arteriole to the smallest venule (vein).

Capillaries permit materials to be exchanged between the blood and tissues. Oxygen and nutrients easily diffuse through the capillary wall. The thin walls of the capillaries are rather like tea-bags, so that the nutrients and oxygen carrying fluid flows on to cells.

Red blood cells

Red blood cells carry the oxygen content of our blood, if we are deficient in red blood cells, we would suffer from anaemia, which if left untreated would cause us to tire easily and would also create a strain on our heart.

Without a nucleus and other organelles, the life span of a red blood cell is about 120 days. New cells are replaced every second, as an old cell dies; this ensures that sufficient red blood cells are produced to carry a constant supply of oxygenated blood.

2 Circulation

The two largest veins of the body are the superior and inferior venae cavae. They empty their contents into the right atrium. This blood passes via the right atrioventricular valve (tricuspid valve) into the right ventricle; from there it is pumped into the pulmonary artery, the only artery in the body which carries deoxygenated blood.

The opening of the pulmonary artery is protected by the pulmonary valve. This valve prevents the backflow of blood into the right ventricle when the ventricular muscle relaxes. *See Figure 10.3.*

After leaving the heart the pulmonary artery divides into the left and right pulmonary arteries which carry the venous blood to the lungs. Here the exchange of gases takes place – carbon dioxide is exhaled and oxygen diffuses into the blood.

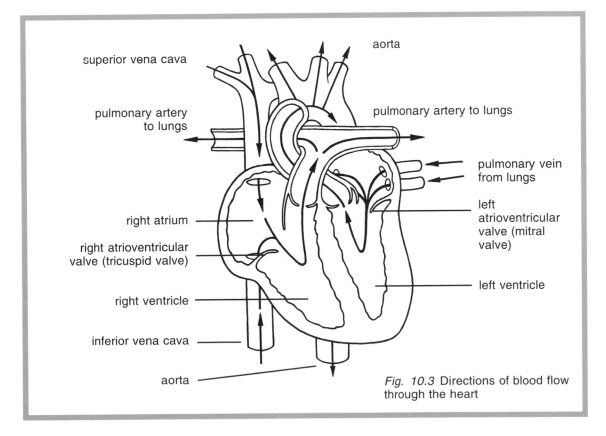

Fig. 10.3 Directions of blood flow through the heart

Two pulmonary veins arising from each lung carry oxygenated blood to the left atrium. Blood then passes through the left atrioventricular valve (bicuspid valve) into the left ventricle and from there it is pumped directly into the aorta which is the largest artery in the body – it is horseshoe in shape. This is the first artery of general circulation and descends behind the heart through the thoracic cavity, a little to the left of the thoracic vertebrae.

At the level of the 12th thoracic vertebrae it passes behind the diaphragm then descends through the abdominal cavity to the level of the 4th lumbar vertebrae. It then divides to form the right and left iliac arteries. The systemic circulation carries blood to the tissues.

The pulmonary circulation consists of the movement of blood from the right ventricle of the heart to the lungs and back to the left atrium.

Coronary heart disease

A disease of affluence, heart disease is a number one killer in the western world today, in fact the statistics are horrifying, as roughly 100,000 men and 70,000 women die from coronary heart disease in the British Isles.

Diet, smoking, an excess of alcohol a sedentary lifestyle and stress are all contributing factors.

If you have a family history of heart disease that also certainly influences your chances of becoming a sufferer and attention to lifestyle changes are even more important.

Coronary heart disease is caused by narrowing of the coronary arteries by atherosclerosis which is the build up of fatty deposits in the artery walls, and just as the corrosion of the internal wall of your water pipe would restrict the flow of water from your tap, exactly the same problem occurs in the arteries to the heart. The myocardium is then deprived of sufficient blood to perform its many functions.

Not only does the heart receive insufficient blood, it cannot get rid of its waste products, and so pain and discomfort are experienced, either in the chest, neck, the arm or sometimes around the bottom of the diaphragm.

When an artery is completely blocked the tissues it supplies rapidly undergo degeneration and die from ischaemia.

The word angina simply means 'chest pain' and is a symptom rather than a condition. The angina will often be caused by very cold weather, exercising after a heavy meal and strong emotions.

Coronary heart disease in men is generally three to six times higher than women, who have some added protection due to the female hormone oestrogen which offers the artery walls a considerable measure of protection. This hormone also assists in avoiding hardening of the peripheral arteries.

Despite the protection from oestrogen, the gap is narrowing as more and more women smoke and drink too much and also are entering the fields of management and professional occupations where their stress levels are ultimately increased.

Blood pressure is determined by the force at which the blood flows through the arteries, the elasticity of the arteries in sustaining the pressure, and the volume of blood in the body. A haemorrhage would lower the pressure whereas poor renal function would raise it.

A clot can form in the arteries if some of the fatty deposits become detached from the artery wall, this would cause an obstruction in the blood flow, depriving the heart of its fuel.

A stroke is a haemorrhage in the brain, a break in a weakened artery, which has been under considerable pressure for years, normally as the result of hypertension. Unfortunately, high blood pressure can remain undetected for many years and is frequently referred to as 'the silent killer'.

An aneurysm is an abnormal swelling in a weakened arterial wall. This may be due to injury or sometimes disease, the weakness is often congenital. It may rupture and haemorrhage will occur.

Back conditions and heart problems

In his book, *The Heart Revolution*, Dr. Paul Sherwood discusses the strong link with back conditions and heart problems, and this has been a very welcomed finding for me personally, for during my long years as a practitioner, and having been involved in treating heart conditions on many occasions, I have been confused when finding such intense sensitivity in the thoracic spine in those suffering from angina, coronary artery disease and the like.

There have been many occasions when people have been admitted into hospital after suffering from a massive heart attack, when tests, even ECGs have been completely normal.

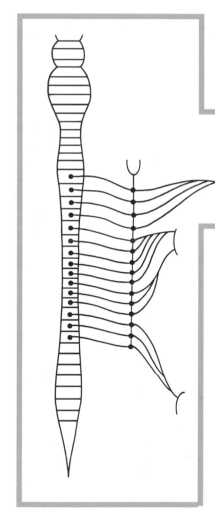

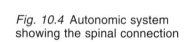

Fig. 10.4 Autonomic system showing the spinal connection

If a clot had caused the coronary blockage it would still be present shutting off the blood supply to the heart muscle, which would ultimately cause much damage. When a muscle is damaged some of it dies and the infarction causes filaments from the dead muscle to be released into the blood stream as proteinous deposits. The reason for the cause of the attack must have been due to a spasm in the coronary artery caused by inflammations and tensions in the muscles, nerves and ligaments in the thoracic and cervical spinal areas. *See Figure 10.4.*

As 'Structure Governs Function' it is not difficult to understand how a long term back condition could be the cause of many heart attacks: the attack not being caused by diseased arteries alone but by muscular spasms. On examining the thoracic and spinal areas in a study of patients who had suffered one or more heart attacks, there was evidence of considerable tension in the paravertebral muscles in the area.

Conditions benefiting from reflexology.

The types of conditions benefiting from reflexology are angina, irregular heart beat, known as tachycardia in its over-productive form and bradycardia in its latent form. Reflexology is also very beneficial for those who have suffered a heart attack. It can be of great support in the postoperative care of these patients.

Any form of circulatory malfunction can be improved with reflexology. Many patients report an improvement in circulation generally and cold feet often become a thing of the past. There are absolutely no dangers associated in treating heart conditions. If you accept that the heart is a muscle that is similar to other organs and muscles in the body, then this becomes a very safe, effective area to work on.

Reflexology benefits the health of diabetic sufferers who have increased problems with circulatory disease during their later years. It is quite normal for a diabetic eventually to suffer coronary conditions. They are more likely to have a stroke, renal failure, loss of sight: unfortunately the blood supply to their legs is often severely diminished and many suffer the disasters of ulceration and gangrene.

Reflexology is of great value to these sufferers and is highly recommended for diabetics of all age groups.

Nutritional help for heart disease

Carnitine, a vitamin-like compound, stimulates the breakdown of long chain fatty acids by the mitochondria which are energy producing units in the cells. Clinical trials have demonstrated that carnitine improves angina and heart disease.

Magnesium deficiency plays a major role in some cases of angina and a magnesium deficiency has been shown to produce spasms of the coronary arteries.

Hawthorn berries offer benefits in the treatment of angina as they help dilate the arteries.

The heart: the symbolism and the reality

I always find it strange that the heart is identified as an organ of romance. Hearts are portrayed on cards expressing feelings for our loved ones; we suffer a broken heart; we have heartfelt warm feelings towards our friends and relatives; we meet many cold hearted people; and we are all aware of the stimulation of heart beat when we experience an emotional response to another person.

If we look at the physical heart it shows nothing of any sentimental or attractive value. It is in fact just a large pump with lots of tubes arising out of it.

Feelings we experience that we associate with our heart in times of happiness or grief are actually vibrations and stimulations from our solar plexus, which is a large nerve complexity behind the stomach. The stimulations and vibrations felt in our heart are due to an increased output of adrenaline, which stimulates heart beat.

Areas to work for heart conditions

In heart conditions, the main areas to work in order to assist the patient are obviously the heart and the lung area. Diaphragm relaxation is of the utmost importance. It is also of great benefit to work the whole of the thoracic spine many times in order to stimulate the nerve supply to the whole thoracic cavity area. Working on the liver is also very beneficial.

CHAPTER 11 Practical procedures for working the circulatory system

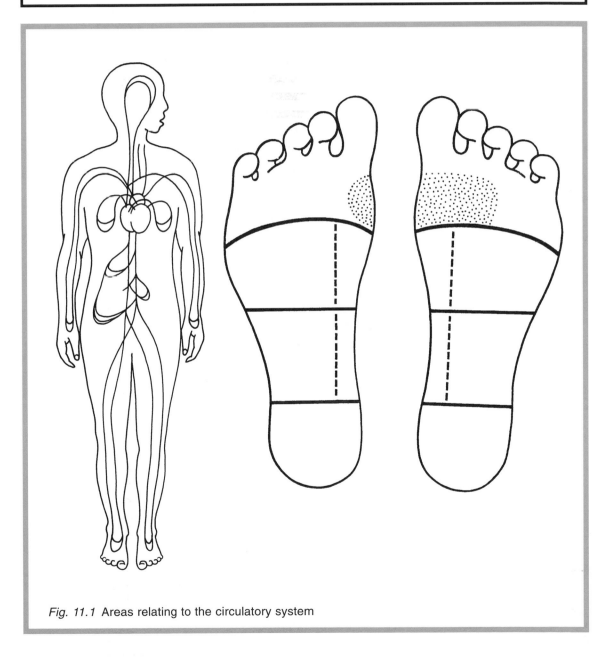

Fig. 11.1 Areas relating to the circulatory system

1 The heart area – *left foot* Zones 1 2 3

1 LEFT FOOT – PLANTAR
MEDIAL TO LATERAL – TOP
SUPPORT

Figure 11.2 Supporting the left foot with your right hand at the top and using the left thumb, work in horizontal lines across the foot from medial to lateral. As the heart will already have been worked out thoroughly within the respiratory area, we do not overwork this area and, therefore, need only to proceed in one direction.

Note Just as organs and functions overlap in the human body, so do reflex points overlap.

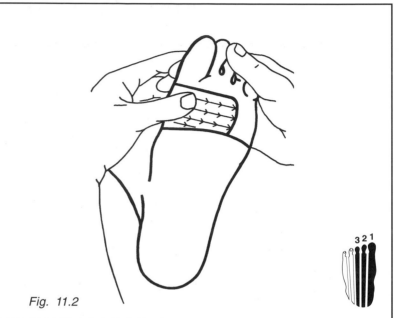

Fig. 11.2

CHAPTER **12** The lymphatic system – a secondary circulatory system

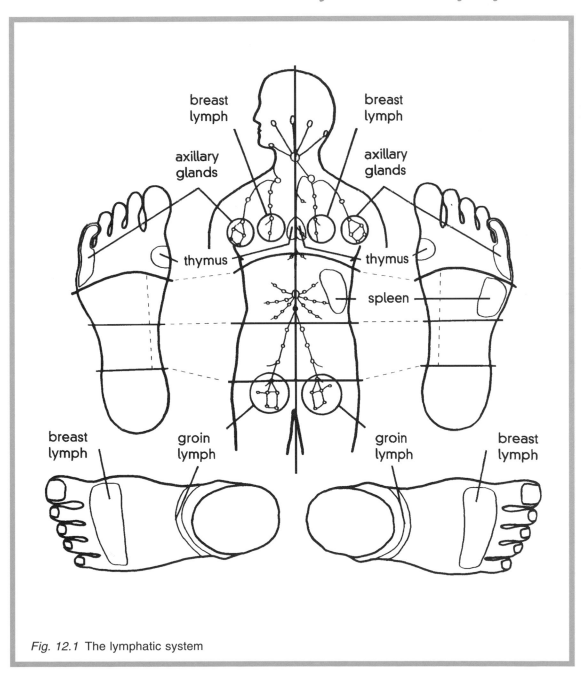

Fig. 12.1 The lymphatic system

THE LYMPHATIC SYSTEM

See Figure 12.1. The lymphatic system is a network of vessels throughout the body that returns tissue fluid to the blood and in this way it helps maintain fluid balance. It also defends the body against disease by producing lymphocytes (a type of white blood cell), and absorbs lipids (fat) from the intestine and transports them to the blood.

The system works by blood pressure forcing fluid from the blood through the capillary wall into surrounding tissues. Most fluids find their way back into the blood vessels, but some enter the initial lymph vessels. The fluid, now called lymph, flows towards the thoracic duct or to the right lymphatic duct.The forces that drive it are muscle activity, pulsation of arteries, the pressure difference in the thorax created by breathing, peristaltic movements of the intestine and contraction of lymph vessels. Valves in lymph vessels ensure that the lymph travels in only one direction.

From the thoracic duct, lymph drains back into the left subclavian vein near the left shoulder.

From the right lymphatic duct, lymph drains back into the right subclavian vein near the right shoulder.

1 Lymph

Lymph is a clear, watery fluid forming in the tissues of the body and normally draining back into the blood circulation. Interstitial fluid is not called lymph until it drains into the network of initial lymph vessels located in the tissue spaces.

The lymphatic system is therefore like a stream of rivers and tributaries. Instead of water, all contain lymph, a salty straw coloured liquid like the fluid part of blood, but with less protein. The system produces tiny vessels which join to form a few larger ones.

2 Lymph vessels – lymphatic ducts

The outer walls of lymph vessels are about the same thickness as small veins. Lymph vessels have many cup-shaped valves which ensures that the lymphatic fluid flows in one direction only, i.e. towards the thorax.

Lymphatic fluid is not pumped like the heart, but it is encouraged by the onward movement of the muscle tissue in the walls of the lymphatic vessels. Movement of lymph is also stimulated by movement i.e. walking, in particular.

Lymphatic vessels return the excess fluid black to the blood, about three litres daily. It returns the plasma protein to the blood.

Fat that is absorbed in the small intestine enters the lymphatic vessels, called lacteals, which transports this milky fluid called chyle, back to the thoracic duct. The thoracic duct is the largest of all and runs up the body in front of the spine. Lymphatic vessels from all over the body, except the upper right quadrant, drain into the thoracic duct. Lymph from the lymphatic vessels in the upper right quadrant of the body drain into the right lymphatic duct.

3 Lymph nodes

Some lymph nodes are the size of a pin head, others the size of an olive: their function is to filter lymph.

When infection invades the body, the lymph nodes swell at strategic points, i.e. the neck, armpit, liver, intestines, groin and knee. The nodes act as an army of defence, as they contain lymphocytes and other white blood cells which fight off any invading bacteria.

As an example, if you have an acute attack of tonsillitis, the lymph nodes around your neck and throat swell in an attempt to prevent the infection arising further into the brain, which is one part of the human body that does not react very favourably to any high increase in temperature. Illnesses that may arise as the result of an infection in the brain are, meningitis, or a 'fit'. Both these conditions are serious and can leave lasting damage. The tonsils are a defence mechanism in the body; the appendix yet another.

4 The spleen

See Figure 12.2. This organ is the largest in the lymphatic system and plays a part in circulation and combating infection. The spleen is a spongy fist sized, purplish

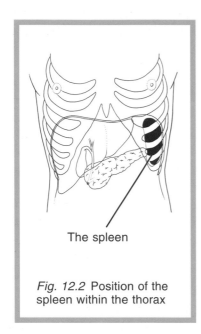

The spleen

Fig. 12.2 Position of the spleen within the thorax

object located just in front of the spine, below the diaphragm and left of and behind the stomach.

The structures entering and leaving the spleen are the splenic artery, splenic vein, lymphatic vessels and nerves

The spleen manufactures some of the blood formed in the body before birth.

As blood flows through the spleen, worn-out red and white blood cells are removed by large scavenger cells, and bacteria and parasites are destroyed. The spleen also produces antibodies and protein to attack viruses and other agents of infection.

5 The thymus gland

This gland, located in the upper thorax, plays a key role in the body's immune process. The gland also secretes the hormone thymosin.

The body's immune system

A healthy body can defend itself against most invading types of organisms that may cause disease.

Unfortunately there are many aspects in our everyday, modern living that cause the lymphatic system to become depressed. The constant use of antibiotics for nearly everything, reduces the effectiveness of the immune system.

Vaccinations have a drastic effect on immunity. Children were meant to get the usual childhood infections: measles, mumps, chicken pox, rubella, whooping cough. These illnesses stimulated the immune system to cope with disease and encourage the spleen to work efficiently in producing white blood cells, lymphocytes, which gave a lifelong protection against disease.

Nonspecific and specific defence mechanisms

There are two types of body defence systems: nonspecific and specific.

Nonspecific defence mechanisms

The following are some important nonspecific defence

mechanisms. The skin is the body's first line of defence against bacteria and other harmful substances. Bacteria which enter the body with inhaled air may be filtered out by the hairs in the nose or trapped in the mucous lining of the respiratory passages or, if they enter with food, the acid and enzymes in the stomach will destroy them. When bacteria invade tissue, inflammation occurs. Nonspecific defence mechanisms operate rapidly.

Specific defence mechanisms

Specific defence is the job of the lymphatic system and is based on specialized white blood cells, the lymphocytes, which respond to invasion of the body by micro-organisms. Lymphocyte B cells produce protein compounds called antibodies. Lymphocyte T cells attack the organism directly.

Artifical immunity – vaccinations

Chemically produced vaccinations do not give life long support; they are also responsible for many other problems in our life today – behavioural problems, i.e. autism, dyslexia, hyperactive children and asthma. Research from experts who are involved in the holistic approach to health – the naturopaths, the herbalists, those involved with the body as a dynamic integrated organism – shows that drugs taken for one disease have an ultimate disastrous effect on another prime function.

Why is it that all these emotional illnesses in children have increased so dramatically in the last thirty years? The reason is that more and more drugs and vaccinations are being used.

Why is the incidence of leukaemia in children increasing? Could it be that the immune system is being so depressed by vaccinations and antibiotics that when a cancer cell appears on the scene, the immune system just does not know what to do with it!

Never before have we had so much terminal disease, no sooner does research provide a control for one disease with drug treatment, than another disease, equally as disastrous as the previous one, takes its place. If only we could pour the billions of pounds of money spent on research into disease into treatment to help the immune system; into the education of our youngsters; into working towards preventing disease by better knowledge of life supports; into diet, exercise, better communications and an understanding of how the mind influences the body, we would prevent many diseases ever occurring. Our mental state and the way we think and behave affects our body so dramatically: our bodies feel our mental pain.

Surely prevention must be a far better way than looking for ever more treatments to relieve disease.

Drugs and the immune system

Unfortunately the drug industry is so very lucrative and good health does not provide profitability.

The future for mankind, as far as the drug industry is concerned is that we will all be encouraged to take more and more drugs for more and more diseases, plus extra medication to take on a regular basis to prevent diseases occurring. In the end our immune system will fail altogether.

We will never be without diseases, they are an integral part of life, but we can do much to help ourselves, if we make the effort to be responsible for what we as an individual do to our own body.

Areas to work to help the lymphatic system

See Figure 12.3. As the lymphatic system is distributed throughout the body, we do not need to isolate, on the feet, specific areas to help the lymphatic system, as we are in fact working out all these areas as we work on the entire body with reflexology.

However, in order to stimulate the thoracic duct which runs in front of the spine in the rib cage area, by working out this area of the spine we would be assisting drainage of the lymphatic system.

Scattered lymph nodes are found under armpits, in intestines and in breast and groin areas.

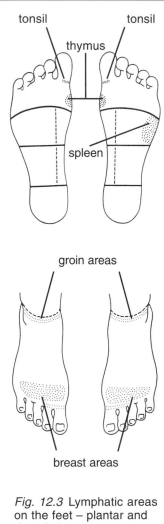

Fig. 12.3 Lymphatic areas on the feet – plantar and dorsal views

CHAPTER 13 The endocrine system

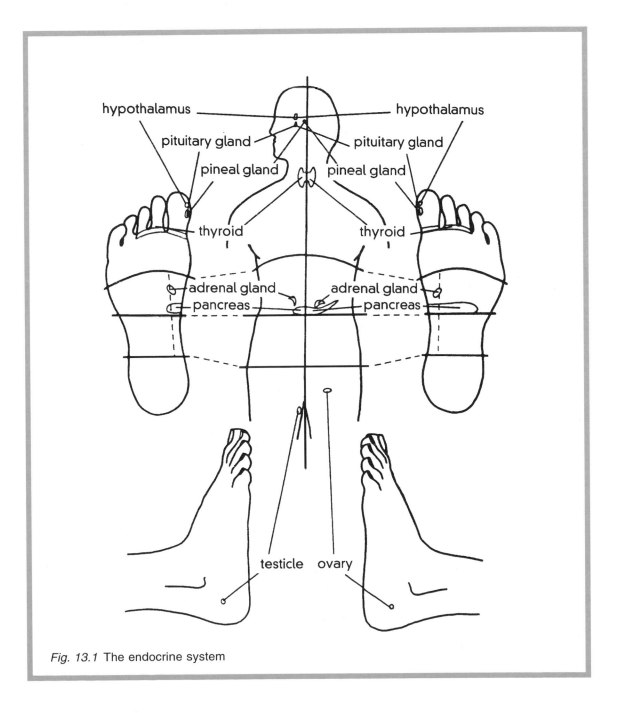

Fig. 13.1 The endocrine system

THE ENDOCRINE SYSTEM

The endocrine system works with the nervous system to maintain a steady state of the body. The functions of the endocrine system include metabolism, use of nutrients by cells, salt and fluid balance, growth, reproduction and helping the body to cope in times of stress. It consists of glands and tissues that release hormones.

The endocrine glands are the hypothalamus, pituitary, the thyroid, four parathyroids, two adrenal glands, the Islets of Langerhans in the pancreas, the pineal gland and two ovaries in the female and the testes in the male, described in Chapter 24.

Hormones are chemical messengers that carry information concerning the speed at which glands and organs work. Hormones are themselves mostly controlled by a mechanism called 'feedback'. When a gland is working overtime, the hormonal system reduces the power, rather like a thermostat. If the activity of a gland becomes sluggish and malfunctions the hormonal system gives it a boost and increases the power.

1 The pituitary gland and the hypothalamus

See Figure 13.2. Endocrine activity is controlled by the hypothalamus. The hypothalamus and pituitary gland act as one unit. The hypothalamus has a direct controlling effect on the pituitary gland and an indirect effect on many others: it links the nervous and endocrine systems.

The pituitary gland regulates the activity of most of the other endocrine glands and is referred to as 'master of the orchestra'. The gland lies between the eyes and behind the nose, and is protected by a very strong arch of bone called the sella turcica (or Turkish saddle).

The following hormones are secreted by the anterior lobe of the pituitary gland:

i) Thyroid stimulating hormone (TSH) Tropic hormones stimulate other endocrine glands. TSH is one such hormone – it activates the thyroid gland.

ii) Adrenocorticotropic hormone (ACTH) is also a tropic hormone which stimulates the adrenal glands.

iii) Gonadotropic hormones are tropic hormones which stimulate gonad function. There are two hormones: follicle stimulating hormone (FSH) and leuteinizing hormone (LH).

FSH stimulates the development and ripening of the ovarian follicle. During its development, the ovarian follicle secretes its own hormone, oestrogen. As the level of oestrogen increases in the blood, so FSH secretion is reduced. The leuteinizing hormone promotes a final maturation of the ovarian follicle and ovulation. Its main function is to promote the formation of the corpus luteum which secretes a second ovarian hormone, progesterone. The follicle stimulating hormone in the male stimulates the epithelial tissue of the seminiferous tubules in the testes to produce spermatozoa. The leuteinizing hormone stimulates the interstitial cells in the testes to secrete the hormone, testosterone.

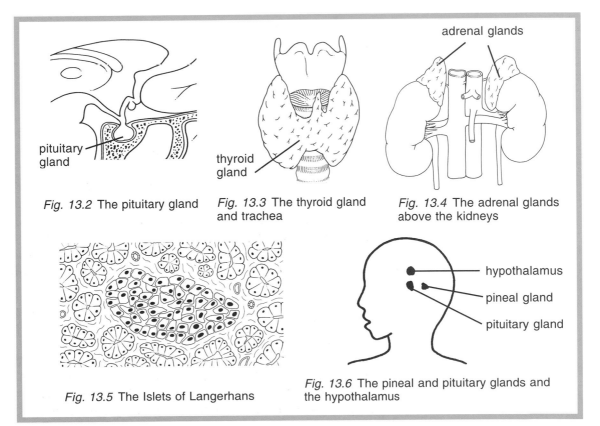

Fig. 13.2 The pituitary gland

Fig. 13.3 The thyroid gland and trachea

Fig. 13.4 The adrenal glands above the kidneys

Fig. 13.5 The Islets of Langerhans

Fig. 13.6 The pineal and pituitary glands and the hypothalamus

iv) Growth hormone (GH) promotes growth of the skeleton, muscles, connective tissue and organs. It is *not* a tropic hormone.

v) Prolactin, during lactation, stimulates the cells of the mammary glands to secrete milk. It is *not* a tropic hormone.

Two other hormones are secreted by the hypothalamus and stored in the posterior lobe of the pituitary and released when required:

vi) Oxytocin promotes contraction of uterine muscles and contraction of the cells of the lactating breast, squeezing milk into the large ducts behind the nipple. In late pregnancy the uterus becomes very sensitive to oxytocin. The amount secreted will be increased just before and during labour as well as when suckling.

vii) Antidiuretic hormone (ADH) regulates fluid balance in the body and indirectly controls blood pressure. ADH helps the body conserve water by increasing water reabsorption from the collecting ducts in the kidneys.

2 The thyroid and parathyroid glands

See Figure 13.3. The thyroid stimulates growth and development and lowers blood calcium level when necessary. It secretes the hormones thyroxine and calcitonin.

The thyroid is responsible for the metabolism of the body and for the extraction of iodine from the blood plasma which has a significant influence on the mental health of individuals. Without iodine the gland cannot make thyroid hormones.

It also influences the heart rate; an overactive thyroid would give you unpleasant palpitations. The heart produces a hormone called atriopeptin which reduces blood volume and blood pressure and so helps to regulate fluid balance.

Apart from the unpleasant palpitations which are experienced when the thyroid gland is overactive, skin and hair would become greasy and anxiety levels would increase with an enlarged appetite but with a paradoxical loss of weight. Insomnia would become a problem. Your body is running in a very high gear, so the ability to relax would be impossible.

If the thyroid gland is underactive there would be an increase in weight, the skin would become dry and scaly, the hair thin and dry and mental abilities would become very reduced. In fact, a child born with a malfunction of the thyroid would be mentally retarded.

The parathyroid glands lie embedded in the thyroid gland and secrete parathyroid hormone, a small protein which regulates the calcium level of the blood and tissue fluid.

The thyroid and parathyroids work together to adjust the blood-calcium level.

3 The adrenal glands

See Figure 13.4. The adrenal glands are found above the kidneys. The inner medulla and outer cortex of the adrenal glands secrete several different hormones.

The medulla secretes epinephrine (adrenalin) and norepinephrine (noradrenalin). Both hormones affect the body during stress. Noradrenalin raises heart rate and blood pressure.

The cortex secretes mineralocorticoids (aldosterone) which maintain sodium and phosphate balance. Glucocorticoids (cortisol) is also secreted and helps the body cope with stress, inflammatory conditions and controls how the body uses carbohydrates, fat and protein.

In addition, a very small amount of sex hormones is secreted, namely, androgen (masculinizing effect) and oestrogen (feminizing effect). These hormones, released in both sexes, are so small that they have little effect on the body.

4 The Islets of Langerhans

See Figure 13.5. These are the endocrine areas of the pancreas and have been described in detail in The Digestive System, Chapter 6.

5 The pineal gland

See Figure 13.6. This little gland which is situated in the fore-brain resembles a pine cone, hence the name pineal. It is connected to the brain by a short stalk containing nerves, many of which terminate in the hypothalamus. It is about 10 mm long, reddish brown in colour and surrounded by a capsule.

Melatonin

Melatonin is the hormone secreted by the pineal gland. There is some direct association between the pineal gland and moods and behaviour patterns.

There is a link-up between the optic nerve and the pineal gland. Recent investigations in Greenland undertaken by a team of psychologists and psychiatrists studying the behaviour of the Eskimo came to many interesting conclusions.

In certain periods of the year Eskimos have to live in semi-twilight and during this time frequently display strange behavioural patterns such as manic depressive states, hysterical and paranoid behaviour and sometimes, in extreme cases, they lose the use of a limb or limbs. This is often referred to as 'hysterical paralysis'.

The psychologists came to the conclusion that these behaviour patterns resulted from the climatic conditions to which the Eskimos were subjected. As a daily routine, treatment was administered by ultraviolet ray into the area where the pineal gland is situated. The results were outstanding; most had treatment by this process for 20 minute sessions every day over the period of a month and 90 per cent of sufferers regained their normal mental state. It is now felt that the pineal gland has some reflecting effect upon the brain which is transmitted via the optic nerve.

Melatonin which is produced by the pineal gland is activated as day light draws to an end. That is why we usually feel sleepy in the late evening. As day light arrives, our pineal gland, is stimulated by light which encourages us to awaken from sleep.

We all know of the seasonal affective disorder commonly referred to as the SAD disease which is quite common in England and many other cold countries. Many people find that during the autumn and winter months they tend to mimic the behavioural pattern of animals. They gain body weight, tend to become less active, sitting about more and find that their mental activities become reduced. This behavioural change continues until spring when the earth and life itself become vital again, light hours lengthen and the symptoms of seasonal affective disorder subside.

The main reasons for these depressive symptoms is lack of sunlight. Ultraviolet light seems to have a direct effect on mood and in some way is absorbed via the eyes to the brain. Although most of us would agree that it is far better to look out on a sunny day than a grey dismal one, you will now understand that it is not just an emotional response, but is in fact a basic physiological problem: we do need sun to keep us in good mental health.

That is probably the reason why the intake into psychiatric hospitals during the autumn and winter months is so high – a starvation of sunlight. It is therefore not surprising to find great sensitivity in the big toe area for those suffering from depression, anxiety and other stress related conditions.

Conditions benefiting from reflexology

Stress and the endocrine system are closely linked therefore the conditions in which we are going to achieve the best results are tension states.

Stress is in the main not destructive; in fact we all need to be stressed at times to be able to achieve anything. It is how the body copes with stress that is all important. Some individuals thrive on stressful situations. In fact they often go through life creating situations to activate stress levels in the body, because they perform better when in an emotionally high powered state. It is when we are tense all the time that troubles in our health begin. In this situation many people exhibit symptoms of illness, such as migraine, indigestion, angina, colitis, asthma, back pain to name but a few. We hold tension in our neck and shoulders.

How often have you said, 'He's a real pain in the neck' when describing a person who created in you bad, unsettled feelings? Our immune system becomes depressed when we are in a tense anxious condition – too much nervous energy has been burnt up and so the general vitality of the body is affected, leaving us wide open for the onset of illness.

People who meditate or practise relaxation techniques regularly get the least disease of all – proof enough that relaxation and good feelings about oneself benefit the body. Racing through life like the speed of light, having little time to 'stand and stare' has a destructive effect.

The greatest benefit we can ever achieve with reflexology is relaxation of body, mind and spirit, the three essentials necessary for the healing process of the body to be set in motion.

Our adrenal glands are active glands which sit on top of each kidney and are very receptive to emotions and feelings. The days when we all lived in caves and caught wild animals to survive have long passed. The release of adrenalin during these times was enormous, as either the wild animal ate us up and that was the end of that, or we killed the beasts and had food for our family for some time.

Tension, anxiety and fright

What actually happens when we are tense, anxious or even frightened? If we relate to the caveman, he stalked his prey, with adrenalin coursing through his veins. He stealthily walked through the jungle, nerves quivering at any movement or sound, his pupils dilated to enable him to see better, his blood was already thickening in his veins so that it would be able to clot faster if he were wounded.

His bronchial tubes dilated to enable him to take in more oxygen, his heart was already beating faster to distribute the oxygen around his body, preparing him to 'run for his life'. He probably had a great desire to urinate frequently or have a bowel movement. I am sure you have often felt the urgent desire to urinate frequently or open your bowels when confronting a situation in your life which made you fearful, such as taking an examination, or confronting an audience to make an after-dinner speech.

That anxiety state is a remnant left from the most primitive forms of life when, to enable you to 'run for your life' you had to be as weightless as possible!

Glucose and fats were being released from the caveman's liver. He needed these elements to give him extra energy and power. Every muscle in his body was vibrating, even his hearing was more acute as he 'listened and watched'.

The wild boar came into view and he ran with his mallet positioned above his head and attacked it. All the energy in his body was stimulated to its peak performance by those two little caps that sit on top of the kidneys – the adrenal glands.

Having killed his prey he tied a rope around the carcass and dragged it back to his cave. The energy used to kill his prey was enormous and after this experience he slept for many hours to recover from the emotional and physical event. This is exactly how the human machine was meant to perform.

However, today we live in a totally different stress-related world. We confront stressful situations all the time because we are living in a fast changing world, with changes that we can hardly keep up with.

If you look back fifty years and list the changes that have occurred in that period, it is incredible. We do not have the anxiety of the wild boar, but we could have a patronising and difficult boss to contend with who releases in us all sorts of emotions from anger to utter despair. We live in fear of redundancy. We fight through traffic jams and worry about the future of our children in a world packed with so much violence.

Our bodies produce the same symptoms and hormones when we experience situations that give rise to anxiety, fear and tension. The big problem is that we never have the opportunity to run for our life or burn off, by extreme physical exercise, the excess of adrenalin. So our body retains the excess of fats, glucose and adrenalin in our veins which just permeate our entire circulatory system, clogging up our arteries and causing all the cardiovascular diseases which are paramount today.

We need more exercise and relaxation, a balance of both. What better way to achieve total relaxation than reflexology? The type of exercise you decide must be up to you.

Generally speaking, reflexology is of great benefit in the relief of menstrual and menopausal discomforts, and it has proved to be of value in helping infertility.

I have had two patients who were unable to conceive due to infrequent ovulation. Within three months both patients conceived and proclaimed the true virtues of reflexology. Many of my practitioners throughout the world have had similar results with many patients.

CHAPTER 14 Practical procedures for working the endocrine system

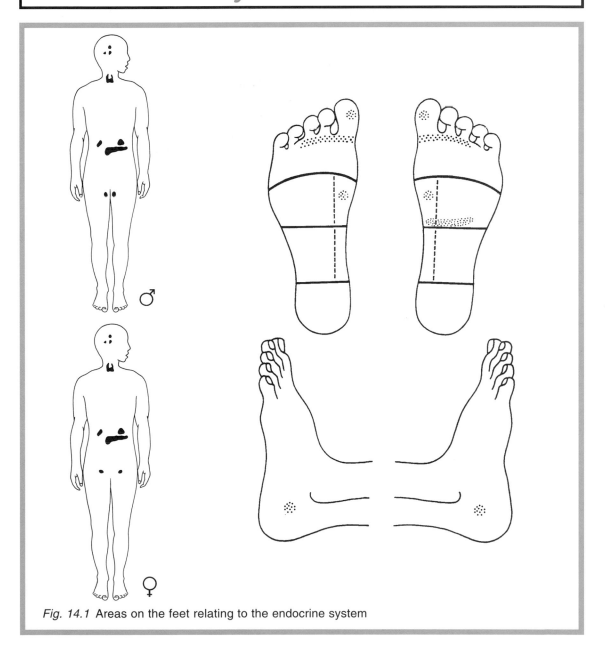

Fig. 14.1 Areas on the feet relating to the endocrine system

1 The pituitary, hypothalamus and pineal areas – *(a) right foot* Zone 1

1 RIGHT FOOT – PLANTAR

MEDIAL – TOP SUPPORT

Figure 14.2 Supporting the right foot at the top with your left hand and using the right thumb, work three times up the medial side of the big toe.

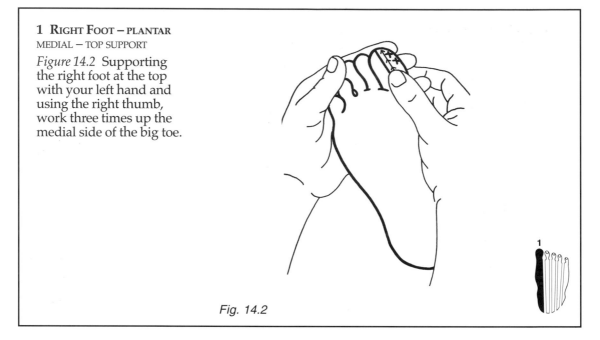

Fig. 14.2

2 The pituitary, hypothalamus and pineal areas – *(b) left foot* Zone 1

1 LEFT FOOT – PLANTAR

MEDIAL – TOP SUPPORT

Figure 14.3 Supporting the left foot at the top with your right hand and using the left thumb, work three times up the medial side of the big toe.

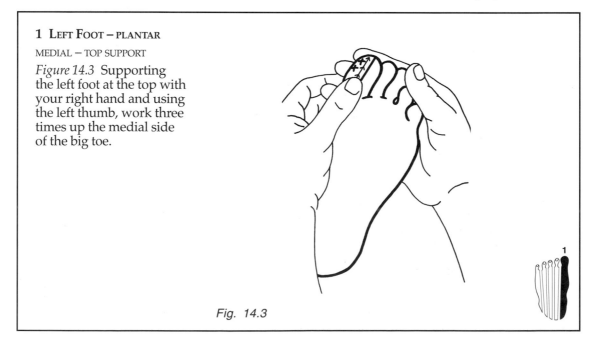

Fig. 14.3

3 The thyroid/neck area – (a) right foot Zones 1 2 3

1 RIGHT FOOT – PLANTAR
MEDIAL TO LATERAL – TOP
SUPPORT

Figure 14.4 Supporting the right foot at the top with your left hand, and using the right thumb, work across the base of the three toes, three times.

2 RIGHT FOOT – DORSAL
MEDIAL TO LATERAL – TOP
SUPPORT

Figure 14.5 Supporting the right foot with your left fist and using the right index finger, work across the join of the toes, three times.

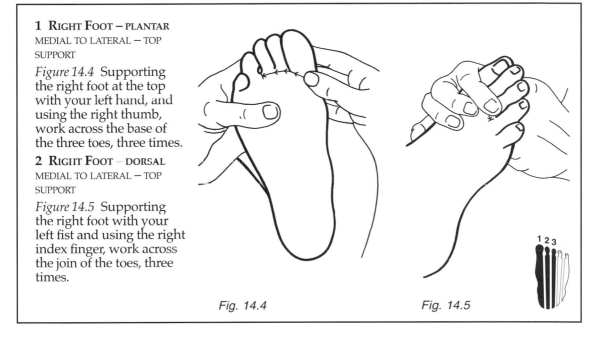

Fig. 14.4   Fig. 14.5

4 The thyroid/neck area – (b) left foot Zones 1 2 3

1 LEFT FOOT – PLANTAR
MEDIAL TO LATERAL – TOP
SUPPORT

Figure 14.6 Supporting the left foot at the top with your right hand, and using the left thumb, work across the base of the three toes, three times.

2 LEFT FOOT – DORSAL
MEDIAL TO LATERAL – TOP
SUPPORT

Figure 14.7 Supporting the left foot with your right fist and using the left index finger, work across the join of the three toes, three times.

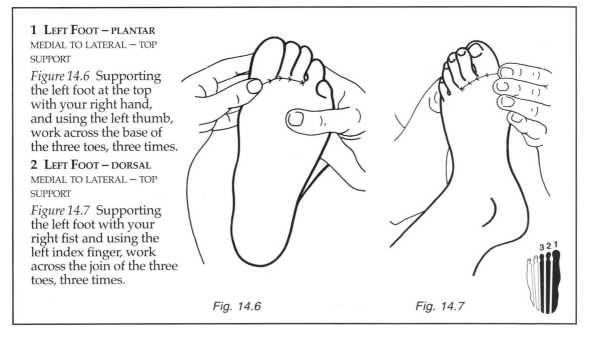

Fig. 14.6   Fig. 14.7

5 The adrenal glands – *(a) right foot* Zone 1

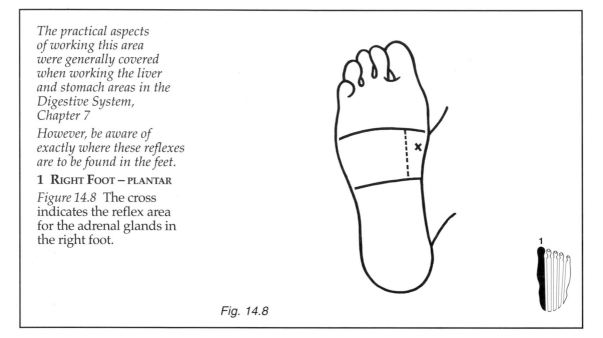

The practical aspects of working this area were generally covered when working the liver and stomach areas in the Digestive System, Chapter 7

However, be aware of exactly where these reflexes are to be found in the feet.

1 RIGHT FOOT – PLANTAR

Figure 14.8 The cross indicates the reflex area for the adrenal glands in the right foot.

Fig. 14.8

6 The adrenal glands – *(b) left foot* Zone 1

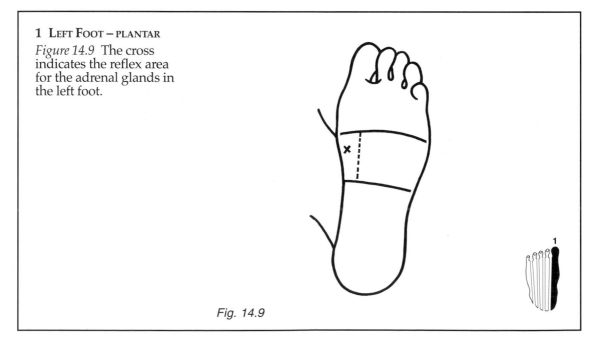

1 LEFT FOOT – PLANTAR

Figure 14.9 The cross indicates the reflex area for the adrenal glands in the left foot.

Fig. 14.9

7 The pancreas – *left foot only* Zones 1 2 3 4

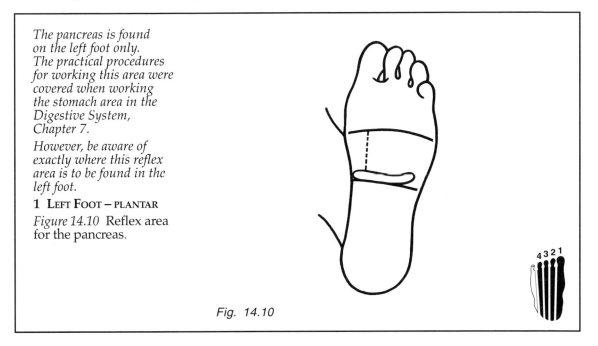

The pancreas is found on the left foot only. The practical procedures for working this area were covered when working the stomach area in the Digestive System, Chapter 7.

However, be aware of exactly where this reflex area is to be found in the left foot.

1 LEFT FOOT – PLANTAR

Figure 14.10 Reflex area for the pancreas.

Fig. 14.10

8 The ovary/testis – *(a) right foot* Zone 5

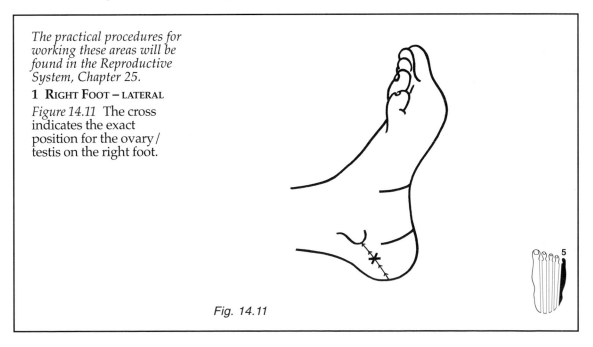

The practical procedures for working these areas will be found in the Reproductive System, Chapter 25.

1 RIGHT FOOT – LATERAL

Figure 14.11 The cross indicates the exact position for the ovary / testis on the right foot.

Fig. 14.11

9 The ovary/testis – (b) left foot Zone 5

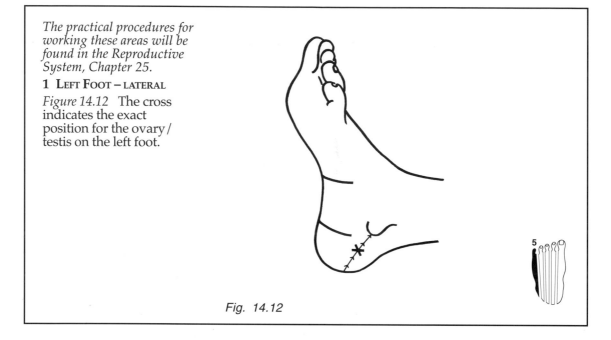

The practical procedures for working these areas will be found in the Reproductive System, Chapter 25.

1 LEFT FOOT – LATERAL

Figure 14.12   The cross indicates the exact position for the ovary / testis on the left foot.

Fig. 14.12

CHAPTER 15 The solar plexus

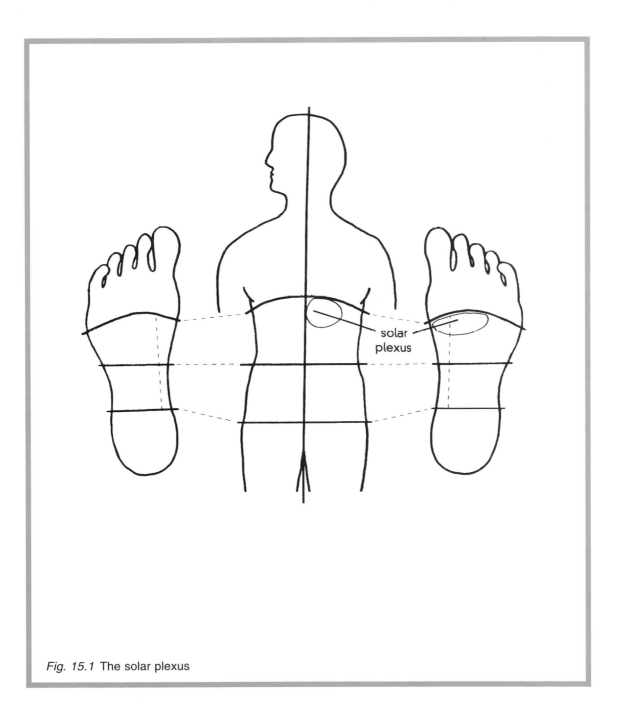

Fig. 15.1 The solar plexus

SOLAR PLEXUS

The solar plexus is a network of nerves which lie behind the stomach wall. 'Solar' is from the word 'sun' and 'plexus' is a grouping together of nerves.

We work on the solar plexus area frequently and automatically as we work on the stomach area, which is on the left side of the body. This is all to the good as it does create a feeling of well-being and has a relaxing effect upon the body.

Generally it is quite usual to pick up sensitivity in this area when treating patients who are under severe emotional strains and pains.

The solar plexus sends out signals in the form of 'butterflies in the stomach' when you are feeling particularly nervous. Maybe there is an impending interview or you have received sad or exciting news about a friend. These strange vibratory signals are all being sent out by our good friend 'the solar plexus'.

Areas to work to help the solar plexus

It is not necessary to work out the area to the solar plexus separately as it lies on the left foot behind the stomach area, just below the diaphragm line, and so it is worked out as one treats the stomach.

However, it is a very good identification of extreme stress in a patient, being almost a barometer to emotional health.

In many instances, pressure applied to this area can result in extreme sensitivity when working with patients who are, perhaps, going through a traumatic period in their lives and are in an anxious condition.

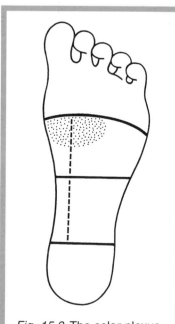

Fig. 15.2 The solar plexus area – plantar view, left foot only.

CHAPTER **16** The nervous system: central and peripheral systems

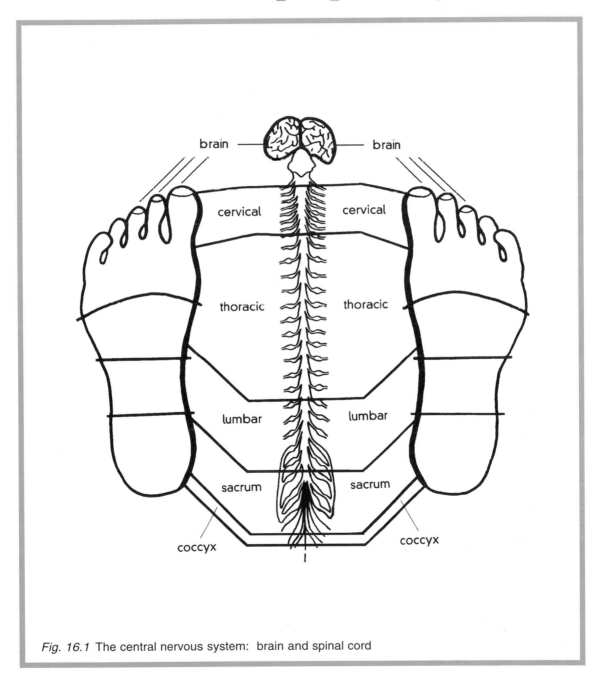

Fig. 16.1 The central nervous system: brain and spinal cord

THE NERVOUS SYSTEM

The nervous system consists of the central nervous system and the peripheral nervous system

The central nervous system

The central nervous system (CNS) comprises the brain and spinal cord.

1 The brain

See Figure 16.2. Located in the skull, the brain looks like a giant wrinkled walnut, crammed inside the skull. The brain contains over 25 billion neurons and supporting glial cells, but weighs less than 1.4 kg (3 lb). With the spinal cord, the brain monitors and regulates many unconscious bodily processes, such as heart rate, and coordinates most voluntary movements.

The brain is the site of consciousness, and all the different intellectual functions which allow human beings to think, learn and create arise from the brain.

It is encased by three connective tissue layers or meninges which contain the cerebrospinal fluid cushioning it against damage. The main parts of the brain are the cerebrum, the cerebellum and the brain stem.

The cerebrum takes up about seven-tenths of the nervous system. It is partially divided into right and left halves, the right and left hemispheres, by a deep groove called the longitudinal fissure. The cerebrum is separated from the cerebellum by the transverse fissure. The brain stem is made up of the medulla, pons and midbrain. Spaces in the brain filled with cerebrospinal fluid are know as ventricles.

The cerebral cortex

The entire area of the cerebrum is covered by a layer of grey matter, the cerebral cortex, beneath which lies the brain's white matter.

The cerebrum

The lobes of the cerebrum specialise in specific functions.

i) The frontal lobe The ability to speak and control voluntary movements of skeletal muscles arise from this part of the brain.

ii) The temporal lobe is concerned with the recognition of sound, emotion, personality and behaviour.

iii) The parietal lobe controls the bodily sensations such as temperature, touch and pain – persons become aware of themselves in relation to their environment.

iv) The occipital lobe detects and interprets visual imagining.

v) The limbic lobe is the ring of cortex and associated structures which surround the ventricles of the cerebrum. It is thought to be a link between emotional and thought processes.

The diencephalon

This part of the brain lies between the cerebrum and midbrain and includes the thalamus and the hypothalamus

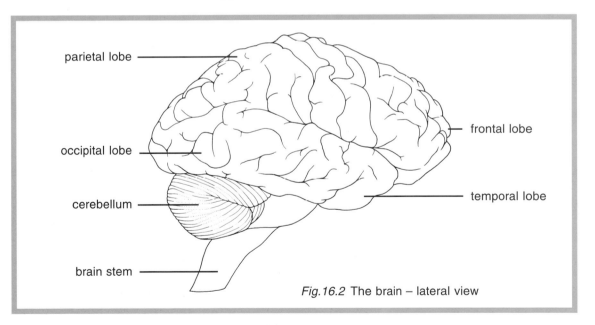

Fig.16.2 The brain – lateral view

The hypothalamus is closely linked with the limbic lobe and has an overall control of autonomic bodily processes.

The thalamus lies in the centre of the brain and acts like an information centre, relaying out important information.

The cerebellum
This is the second largest part of the brain responsible for coordination of movement.

The brain stem
This contains centres that are vital for survival, respiration, blood pressure, heartbeat and digestion.

The skull
The brain is encased in the solid bones of the skull, under which are the meninges which contain cerebrospinal fluid.

Cerebrospinal fluid
This fluid fills the ventricles (the cavities within the brain) and the spaces between the meninges in the brain and spinal cord. The fluid protects and nourishes the brain and spine and, most important of all, it contains lymphocytes that guard the brain against infection, the most dangerous of which is meningitis.

Cerebrospinal fluid consists of mineral salts, water, glucose, plasma proteins, creatinine and urea. Apart from having its protective and nourishing aspects it acts as a cushion and shock absorber between the brain and the cranial bones. It is also useful for analysis when diagnosing diseases such as polio, meningitis and multiple sclerosis.

Cerebrospinal fluid is secreted into each ventricle of the brain by choroid plexuses. These consist of areas where the lining membrane of the ventricle walls is fragile and has quantities of blood capillaries. The fluid passes back into the blood through tiny diverticula of arachnoid matter. The movement of the CSF is secreted continuously at the rate of about 0.5 ml per minute.

The blood supply to the brain
The vascularity of the brain is immense, with blood supplying the arteries, veins and capillaries with this life giving fluid containing both oxygen and glucose. Without these elements brain function deteriorates rapidly. With a lack of oxygen lasting longer than six minutes brain damage or death would result.

Branches of the internal carotid arteries and the basilar artery form a circle of arteries at the base of the brain. This circle is called the circle of Willis and from this point blood vessels provide the brain with oxygenated blood.

A stroke is an eruption of a blood vessel in the brain. This is usually caused in those who have a history of high blood pressure.

The arteries in the brain are not so strong as other arteries in the body and therefore a raised blood pressure will cause an excess strain on blood supply to the brain.

Eventually the constant pressure causes a bulge in the artery wall which bursts and creates a 'bleed in the brain'. Blood fills the cranium causing pressure and inflammation. This in turn affects the nerve supply to the body, resulting in a loss of speech, and usually paralysis of an arm and leg. Most strokes are one sided.

Reflexology has proved to be very successful in helping stroke victims, provided the treatment is given just as soon after the incident as is possible. Treatment on a daily basis must be given in order that the maximum benefit is achieved.

2 The spinal cord

See Figure 16.3. The spinal cord is just like a flex of wire about 43 cm (17 in) in length and descends from the brain stem to the edge of the second lumbar vertebra. It is about as wide as your little finger, and extends from the upper border of the atlas.

31 pairs of spinal nerves arise from the spinal cord and information received from these nerves stimulates impulses throughout the entire human form.

The cord is protected by the bony segments of the vertebral column and meninges.

The spinal cord occupies only the first two thirds of the vertebral column, tapering off to form a tail-like structure which is protected by the sacrum.

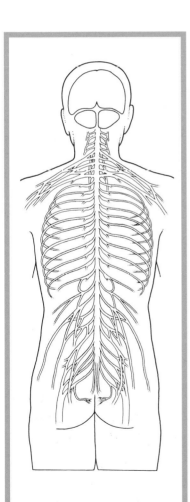

Fig. 16.3 Spinal nerves

The peripheral nervous system

The peripheral nerves convey information both to and from the brain and spinal cord. Sensory nerves receive information from the skin and the internal organs while motor nerves initiate the action of various structures.

The peripheral nervous system (PNS) consists of 12 pairs of cranial nerves from the under the surface of the brain and 31 pairs of spinal nerves from the spinal cord extending out through spaces between the vertebrae.

Let us now take a look at the nerves arising from each part of the spine. *See Figures 16.4 and 32.4.*

Cervical – C1 to C4 cervical plexus and the odontoid peg and C5 to C8 and Thoracic 1 – brachial plexus.
These nerves stimulate the back of the head, the neck, hands and arms as well as the diaphragm muscle which is essential in respiration.

Thoracic nerves – T1 to T12 directly affect the muscles between the ribs which are known as the intercostal muscles which allow the expansion out of the rib cage. Some of the muscles in the back and abdominal regions are also controlled by these nerves.

Lumbar nerves – L1 to L5 and the lumbar plexus
Four of the five pairs of lumbar spinal nerves (L1 to L4) form the lumbar plexus which supplies the low back as well as the sacral area.

Sacral region – S1 to S5 and the sacral plexus
These nerves innervate the thighs, buttocks, the muscles of the skin, legs and feet, the rectum and genital area.

The sacral plexus is formed by nerves **L5 to S3.** The main branch of this plexus is the sciatic nerve.

Coccygeal region The coccygeal plexus is small, formed by **S4 to C1.**

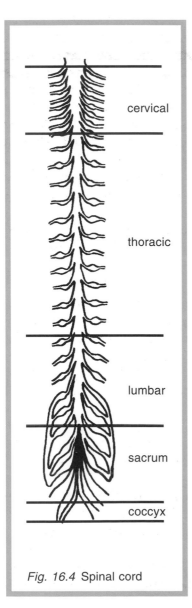

cervical

thoracic

lumbar

sacrum

coccyx

Fig. 16.4 Spinal cord

Spinal nerves

There are 31 pairs of spinal nerves that leave the vertebral canal by passing through the intervetebral foramina formed by adjacent vertebrae.

They are named and grouped according to the vertebrae which they are associated with. We have eight cervical nerves, twelve thoracic, five lumbar, five sacral and one coccygeal.

Although we only have seven cervical vertebrae in our neck, we do in fact have eight nerves, the first pair leaving the vertebral column between the occipital bone and the atlas, and the eighth pair leave below the 7th cervical vertebrae. We therefore give to the nerves the name and number of the vertebrae immediately above.

The coccygeal, sacral and lumbar nerves leave the spinal cord near its termination, i.e. at the level between the first and second lumbar vertebrae and then extend downwards forming a group of nerves which resembles the tail of a horse and commonly known as the cauda equina.

Spinal nerves arise from both sides of the spinal cord and emerge through the intervetebral foramina.

The autonomic nervous system

The autonomic nervous system consists of the peripheral nervous system and works to maintain a steady state within the internal environment of the body. Sensory fibres run through cranial and spinal nerves. The motor portion is divided into sympathetic and parasympathetic systems and are also part of some spinal and cranial nerves.

The sympathetic system prepares the body for action. The parasympathetic system is most active during periods of calm and rest – it conserves and restores energy.

Many organs have both sympathetic and para-sympathetic nerves, e.g. the heart: sympathetic nerves increase the rate and the parasympathetic (vagus) nerves slow it down.

The digestive system is mainly under para-sympathetic control. Whilst food remains in your mouth, you have the freedom of choice to spit it out, or swallow it. Once swallowed the peristaltic muscular contractions take over and force food down through the oesophagus to the stomach.

The vagus nerves

These nerves have more of an extensive distribution than any other cranial nerves, as they arise from nerve cells in the medulla oblongata and pass through the neck into the thorax and the abdomen.

Neorological disorders

Multiple sclerosis, epilepsy, Parkinson's disease, Alzheimer's disease: these are all conditions which affect the nervous system.

It is well worthwhile treating these conditions, particularly in the early stages, and good responses have been obtained.

Paralysis or weakness of various areas in the body result from damage to the motor areas of the brain or nerve pathways of the spinal cord.

As well as damage to the muscle activity which will render the patient unable to move, breathing may also be affected.

In paraplegia the middle or lower area of the spinal cord can cause paralysis of the legs and trunk. Retention of both bladder and bowel function may also be affected and catheterization may be necessary.

Quadriplegia results from damage in the area C1 to T4. If damage occurs between C1 and C2 survival is unlikely.

Hemiplegia causes damage to the motor areas on one side of the brain which causes paralysis to the opposite side of the body.

How reflexology can help

Working the central nervous system and brain is so vital in treating with reflexology. In fact, this is **the** most important area to work in reflexology. If you only had 20 minutes to work on your best friend who, perhaps, was feeling tired, had a bad headache, or menstrual cramps, by working on the central nervous system via the feet you will be stimulating the entire central nervous system.

Remember, nerve impulses arising from the spine serve all organs, functions and parts of the human body, so as you work on the spinal area you are giving this vital stimulation to the whole human form.

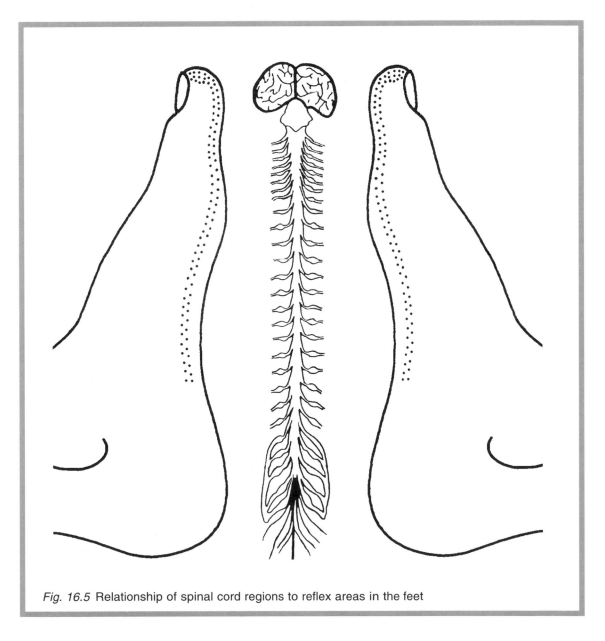

Fig. 16.5 Relationship of spinal cord regions to reflex areas in the feet

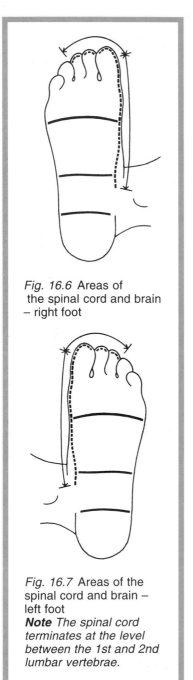

Fig. 16.6 Areas of
the spinal cord and brain
– right foot

Fig. 16.7 Areas of the
spinal cord and brain –
left foot
Note *The spinal cord
terminates at the level
between the 1st and 2nd
lumbar vertebrae.*

Areas to work to help the central nervous system

The central nervous system – spinal column and brain are in Zones 1, 2 and 3. *See Figures 16.6 and 16.7.*

Zone 1 is the most powerful zone in the body as within this zone we have the area for our brain, containing the pituitary, the hypothalamus and pineal area, spinal cord and vertebral column; our naval, which is our very life support before birth, and our reproductive organs, which ensure the continuation of the next generation.

It is not unusual therefore to find that most people have a sensitivity in this zone.

When you are treating people for whatever condition they approach you for, concentrate on working extensively on whichever part of the spinal area supports the ailing part. Constant reference to the information in this chapter will soon acquaint you with an understanding of the nerve supply to specific parts of the body. You will find that your results improve rapidly.

As an example, you would get such outstanding results when treating a patient suffering the effects of a heart attack or angina if you worked out the area of the thoracic spinal nerves, as well as the heart and lung.

Remember, reflexology is not just about working on the spine to help back pain or the intestines to help your constipation, it is having a true understanding of the working of the entire human body, a study of the nerve supply and not only where to contact these delicate structures in the feet, but how to apply the correct pressure and technique to achieve the desired result.

CHAPTER 17 Practical procedures for working the nervous system: central & peripheral systems

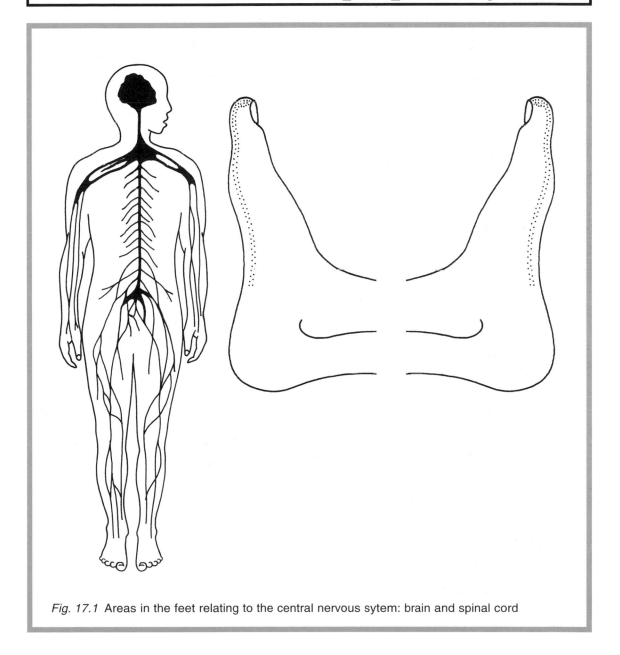

Fig. 17.1 Areas in the feet relating to the central nervous sytem: brain and spinal cord

1 The brain and spinal cord – *(a) right foot* Zones 1 2 3

1 RIGHT FOOT – PLANTAR
TOP SUPPORT

Figure 17.2 Supporting the right foot with your left hand at the top and using the right thumb, work up the spine and into the brain area two or three times.

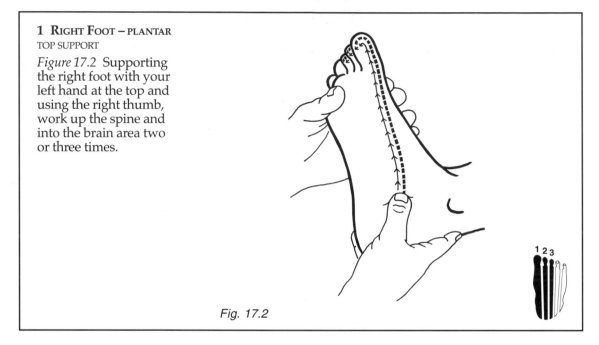

Fig. 17.2

2 The brain and spinal cord – *(b) left foot* Zones 1 2 3

1 LEFT FOOT – PLANTAR
TOP SUPPORT

Figure 17.3 Supporting the left foot with your right hand at the top and using the left thumb, work up the spine and into the brain area two or three times.

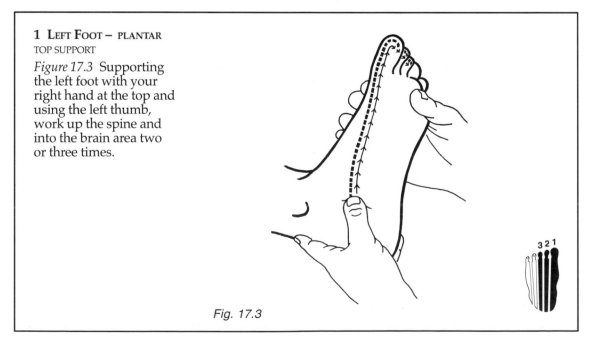

Fig. 17.3

CHAPTER 18 The ear, eye, nose, throat, facial and sinus areas

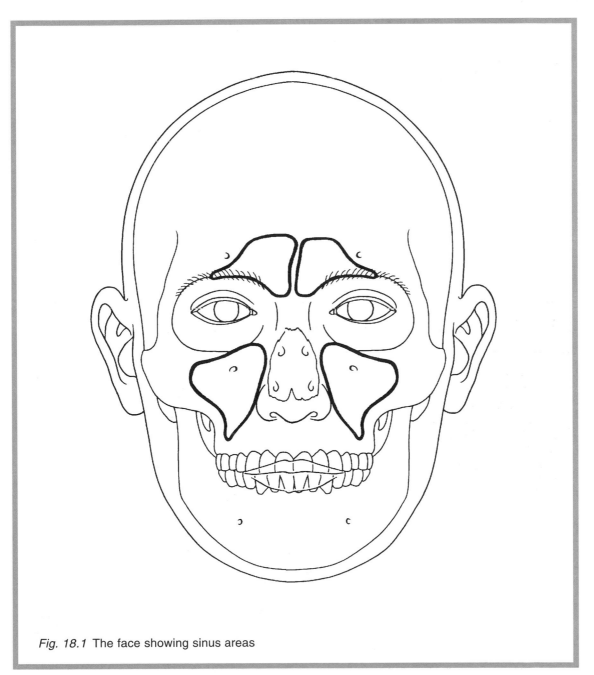

Fig. 18.1 The face showing sinus areas

THE EAR

See Figure 18.2. Ears contain structures that enable us to hear and keep our balance. The human ear is sensitive to sounds ranging in loudness from 10 to 140 decibels (10 million times as loud as 10) and ranging in pitch from 20 to a high of 20,000 hertz cycles per second.

Every sound produces sound waves or vibrations in the air. Sound waves have pitch and volume or intensity. Pitch is determined by the frequency of sound waves. The volume depends on the amplitude of the sound waves which are measured in decibels.

The distance between the ears helps the brain to locate the direction of the sound and its source. The structure of the ears is as follows.

Each ear comprises three parts, the outer ear, the middle ear and the inner ear.

The outer ear

This consists of a cartilage flap, the pinna and the meatus or ear canal.

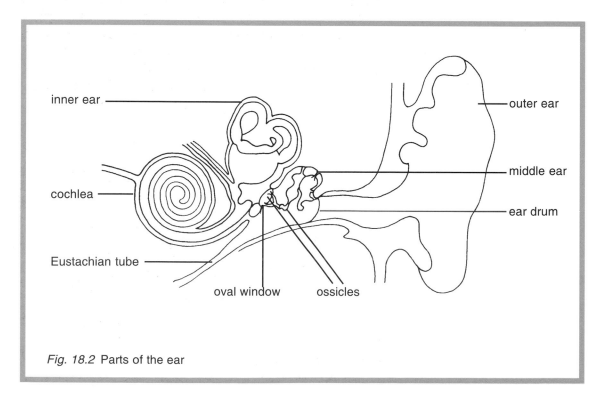

Fig. 18.2 Parts of the ear

The middle ear

See Figure 18.3. The middle ear has an ear drum leading to three tiny bones or ossicles: the malleus (the hammer), incus (anvil), and stapes (stirrup). The Eustachian tube opens into the back of the throat and keeps the middle ear pressure the same as that outside.

The inner ear

A coiled, fluid filled tube, the cochlea, is in the inner ear. This coiled tube really resembles a snails shell. It has a broad base where it is continuous with the vestibule and a narrow apex, with a so-called oval window and round window, containing the organ of Corti with nerve cells connected to the auditory nerve. The organ of balance comprises three fluid filled semicircular canals (U shaped tubes) containing hairs sensitive to movement and cells able to sense bodily positioning.

How hearing works

The pinna funnels send waves through the ear canal where they vibrate the eardrum. The ossicles amplify this vibration and transmit it by the oval window to the fluid in the cochlea. Here, cells in the organ of Corti, interpret vibrations as nerve impulses carried by the auditory nerve to the brain. Meanwhile, vibrations leave the cochlea through the round window.

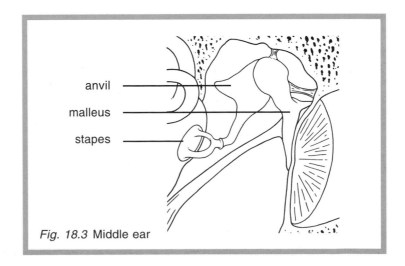

anvil

malleus

stapes

Fig. 18.3 Middle ear

THE EYES

See Figure 18.4. The sclera or white forms the outer layer of the eyeball. The sclera joins the cornea, the transparent layer which covers the iris and pupil, at the front of the eye. The sclera is covered by a thin protective membrane called the conjunctiva which is lubricated by salty fluid secreted by the lachrymal gland on the inside of the upper eyelid.

The iris is the coloured part of the eye made up of smooth muscle tissue. The opening in the centre of the circular muscles of the iris is the pupil.

Behind the cornea lies the anterior chamber of the eye, containing the watery fluid, aqueous humour. This is separated from the posterior chamber by the lens. The posterior chamber contains vitreous humour, a much firmer jelly giving the eyeball its firmness.

Light is admitted through the central black hole, or pupil to the back of the eye through the lens to focus on the retina. The light is focused as it passes through the cornea and aqueous humour.

Inside the eye, light rays from an object are bent by the cornea and lens so that the rays come to focus on the retina. The retina is the innermost layer of the eye and contains sensory receptors called rods and cones which transmit signals through the retina to the optic nerve.

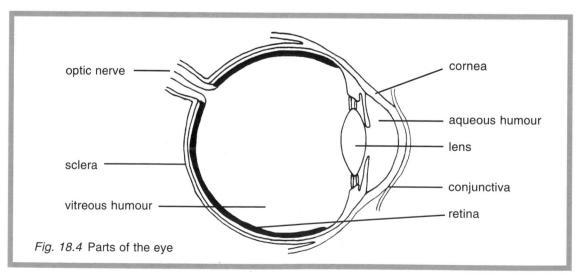

Fig. 18.4 Parts of the eye

SINUS AND FACIAL AREAS

See Figure 18.5. Cells sensitive to smell occur in the olfactory nerves. They have their origins in special cells in the mucus membrane of the roof of the nose, above the superior nasal passage. On each side of the nasal septum nerve fibres from the cells pass through the nasal area.

The sense of smell in human beings is generally less acute than in other animals. All odorous materials give off chemical particles which are carried into the nose and the olfactory region when dissolved in mucus.

When an individual is continuously exposed to an odour, perception of the odour quickly decreases and eventually ceases.

Air entering the nose is heated and convection currents carry eddies of inspired air from the main stream to the roof of the nose. 'Sniffing' concentrates more particles more quickly to the roof of the nose. This increases the number of special cells stimulated and thus the perception of the smell. The sense of smell may affect the appetite. If the odours are pleasant the appetite may improve and vice versa.

Inflammation of the nasal mucosa prevents odorous substances from reaching the olfactory area of the nose causing loss of the sense of smell. The usual cause is the common cold.

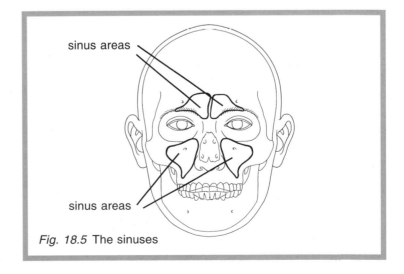

Fig. 18.5 The sinuses

How reflexology can help

The types of conditions reflexologists are able to help relieve are: eye and ear conditions, particularly tinnitus, constant ear, nose and throat conditions in children; tired, strained eyes and conjunctivitis.

If you are suffering from an acute pain due to problems with your teeth, search around the fronts of the three toes and you will find an acute sensitive spot in these areas. If the problem is on the right side of your jaw, the sensitivity will be in the right toes. If the problem occurs on the left side of your jaw, the sensitivity will be found in the left toes.

This will help to relieve the pain before you are to arrange an appointment with your dentist. I must stress that this will only relieve the condition temporarily and professional help must be taken.

The same help can be used if you are suffering from neuralgia or any other form of facial pain.

Many people going through an extremely stressful situation in their lives find that their eyesight deteriorates rapidly. This is caused by tension and when both stress and tension are relieved with reflexology, their eyesight quickly returns to its normal state.

Sinus conditions affect the areas of taste and smell and also cause extreme congestion in the nasal cavities which in turn causes pressure, pain and infection in the facial areas.

Sinusitis is often caused by an infection which comes about after a heavy cold, leaving you with catarrh. Alternatively, it can be complicated by an episode of hay fever, which causes irritation and infection to the linings of the nose and throat. These conditions can easily be relieved by reflexology.

CHAPTER 19 Practical procedures for working the ear, eye, nose, throat, facial and sinus areas

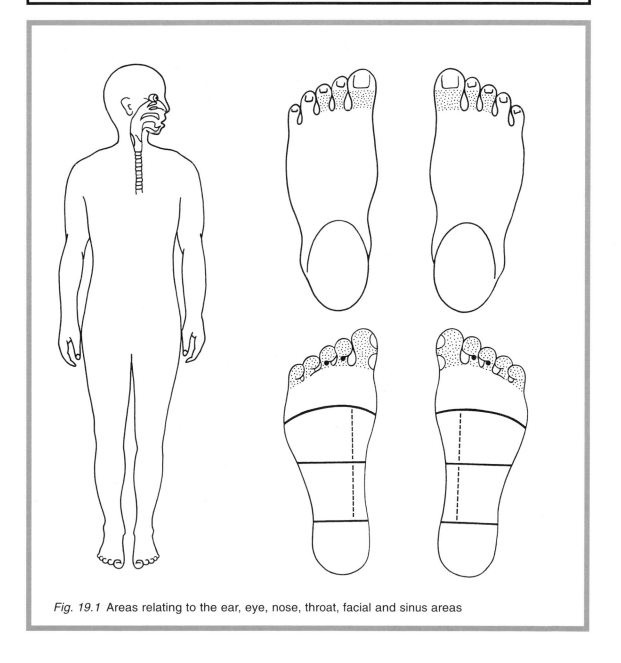

Fig. 19.1 Areas relating to the ear, eye, nose, throat, facial and sinus areas

1 The sinus areas – *(a) right foot* Zones 1 2 3 4 5

1 RIGHT FOOT – PLANTAR
MEDIAL TO LATERAL – TOP
SUPPORT
Figure 19.2 Supporting the right foot with your left hand at the top and using the right thumb, work upwards in straight lines, from medial to lateral.

2 RIGHT FOOT – PLANTAR
LATERAL TO MEDIAL – TOP
SUPPORT
Figure 19.3 Supporting the right foot with your right hand at the top and using the left thumb, work upwards in straight lines, from lateral to medial.

Note The crosses indicate the reflex areas for the nose and throat.

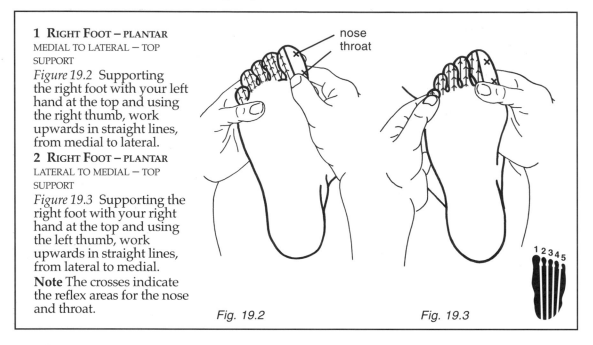

nose
throat

Fig. 19.2   Fig. 19.3

2 The sinus areas – *(b) left foot* Zones 1 2 3 4 5

1 LEFT FOOT – PLANTAR
MEDIAL TO LATERAL – TOP
SUPPORT
Figure 19.4 Supporting the left foot with your right hand at the top and using the left thumb, work upwards in straight lines, from medial to lateral.

2 LEFT FOOT – PLANTAR
LATERAL TO MEDIAL – TOP
SUPPORT
Figure 19.5 Supporting the left foot with your left hand at the top and using the right thumb, work upwards in straight lines, from lateral to medial.

Note The crosses indicate the reflex areas for the nose and throat.

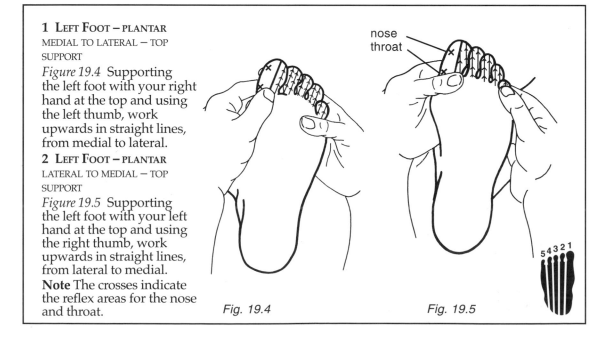

nose
throat

Fig. 19.4   Fig. 19.5

1 The eye and ear areas – (a) right foot Zone 2 & Zone 3

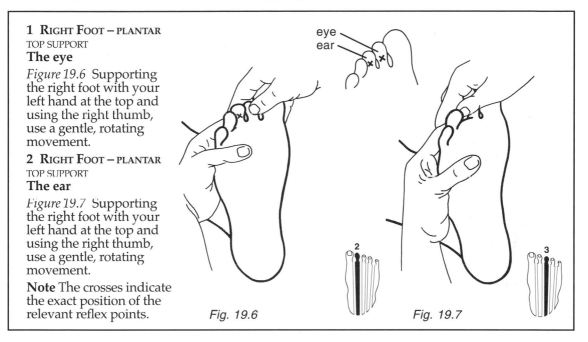

1 RIGHT FOOT – PLANTAR
TOP SUPPORT
The eye

Figure 19.6 Supporting the right foot with your left hand at the top and using the right thumb, use a gentle, rotating movement.

2 RIGHT FOOT – PLANTAR
TOP SUPPORT
The ear

Figure 19.7 Supporting the right foot with your left hand at the top and using the right thumb, use a gentle, rotating movement.

Note The crosses indicate the exact position of the relevant reflex points.

Fig. 19.6   Fig. 19.7

2 The eye and ear areas – (b) left foot Zone 2 & Zone 3

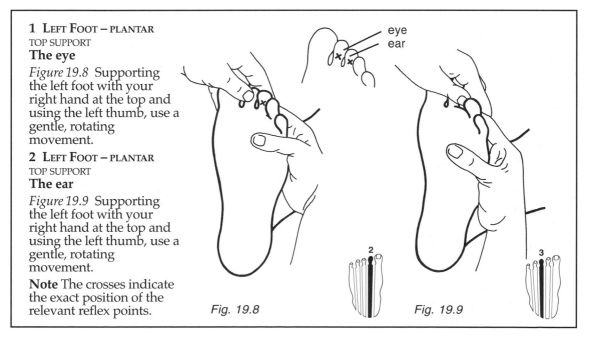

1 LEFT FOOT – PLANTAR
TOP SUPPORT
The eye

Figure 19.8 Supporting the left foot with your right hand at the top and using the left thumb, use a gentle, rotating movement.

2 LEFT FOOT – PLANTAR
TOP SUPPORT
The ear

Figure 19.9 Supporting the left foot with your right hand at the top and using the left thumb, use a gentle, rotating movement.

Note The crosses indicate the exact position of the relevant reflex points.

Fig. 19.8   Fig. 19.9

1 The facial area – *(a) right foot* Zone 1 2 3

1 RIGHT FOOT – DORSAL
MEDIAL TO LATERAL – TOP
SUPPORT

Figure 19.10 Supporting the right foot with your left hand and using the right index finger, work across the first three toes, two or three times, from medial to lateral.

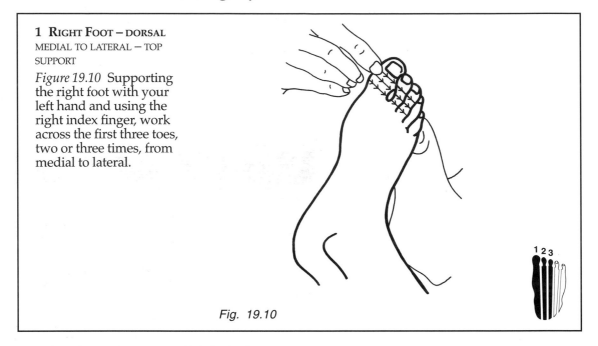

Fig. 19.10

2 The facial area – *(b) left foot* Zone 1 2 3

1 LEFT FOOT – DORSAL
MEDIAL TO LATERAL – TOP
SUPPORT

Figure 19.11 Supporting the left foot with your right hand and using the left index finger, work across the first three toes, two or three times, from medial to lateral.

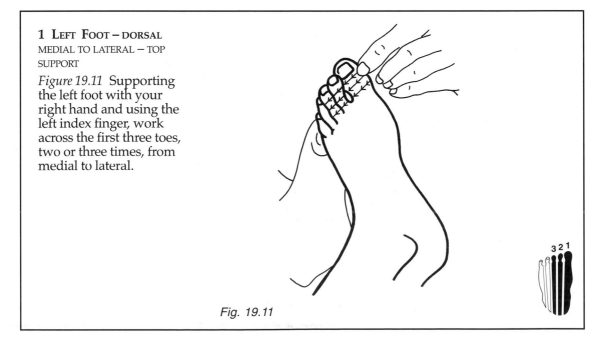

Fig. 19.11

CHAPTER **20** The skeletal and muscular
systems

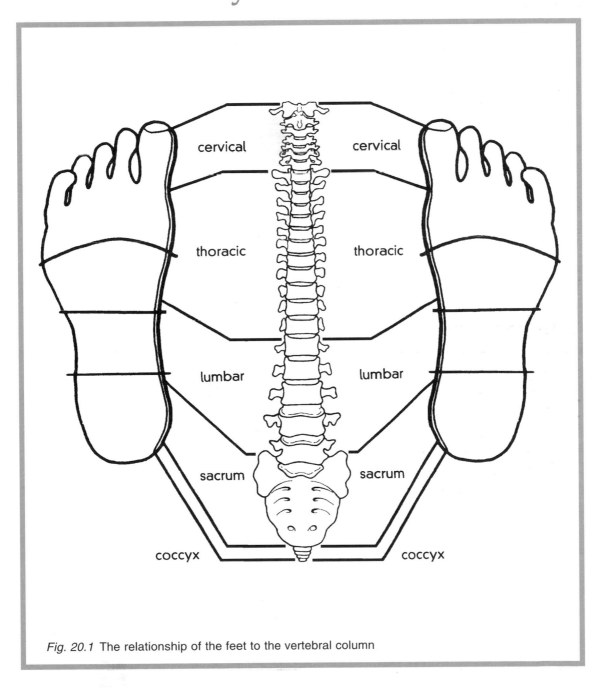

Fig. 20.1 The relationship of the feet to the vertebral column

THE SKELETAL SYSTEM

The living skeleton is a very flexible strong structure, which enables us to move stretch, bend, and rotate our bodies at will.

There is more life in bone than most people believe, and because of the great age people are surviving to today, there is obviously more wear and tear in our bones and joints, and replacement hips, knees and joints in our spine are very usual everyday occurrences in our hospitals.

The skeleton consists of about 206 bones and may be divided into two broad groups: the axial skeleton and the appendicular skeleton. It has five main functions: to provide support, to protect the internal organs, to give movement by using specialised muscles, to produce blood cells and for the storage and release of minerals such as calcium and phosphorous. The axial skeleton consists of the skull, spine and rib cage and sternum supplying the basic structure on to which the appendicular skeleton, the limbs, are joined via the pelvic and shoulder girdles.

The skeleton is built up of certain sets of bones: long bones from hip to knee and from shoulder to elbow; short bones of the fingers and toes; flat bones of the cranium, scapula and sternum area and irregular bones of the spine, pelvic area and stapes in the middle ear.

The pelvic girdle is much stronger than the shoulder girdle as it has to support the full weight of the body.

The spinal column is very much like cotton reels upon a rope, and the spine itself has tremendous abilities for movement. We can bend forwards, backwards, to the right, to the left, rotate our head upon our neck, look downwards to the floor and upwards to the ceiling.

1 Bones

All bones have an outer, compact layer and an inner, spongy centre. This makes them strong and light. They also act as storage for calcium and phosphorus. The articulating surfaces of the bone are covered with hyaline cartilage to supply a smooth surface for the joints. There is no nerve supply to the bone, but blood vessels enter through the nutrient canal to reach the spongy centre. Each bone is covered by a layer of specialised connective tissue called the periosteum.

Growth takes place in all bones, but is more obviously apparent in long bones. During foetal development bones form in two ways. The long bones develop from cartilage and the flat bones of the skull, vertebrae and some other bones develop from a noncartilage connective tissue – membrane.

Bone is a type of connective tissue that is as strong as steel, but still very light. It is made of specialised cells, protein fibres, interwoven into a gel-like substance which is composed of water, salts and carbohydrates. Bones contain bone marrow, a soft tissue that produces blood cells.

As we age our bones become notably more porous and thinner. Osteoporosis is more common in women after the menopause when their supplies of oestrogen diminish. Men also are prone to the calcium loss in bones as testosterone levels decline in later years.

2 Joints

A joint is a meeting point of bones. It usually allows a controlled amount of movement. Some joints have to be very strong; others tend to be very mobile.

The articulating surfaces of bone are covered with smooth hyaline cartilage. A joint has a strong fibrous capsule surrounding the bone ends and has stabilising ligaments which bind and strengthen it. There are different types of joints:

Fibrous joints

These are bones held together by fibrous tissue, e.g. the sutures of the skull.

Cartilaginous joints

The bone ends are covered by hyaline cartilage and between the ends of the hyaline cartilage is a disc of fibrocartilage. These joints are found in the midline of the body, e.g. between the bodies of the vertebrae – intervertebral joints and the symphysis pubis between the pubic bones.

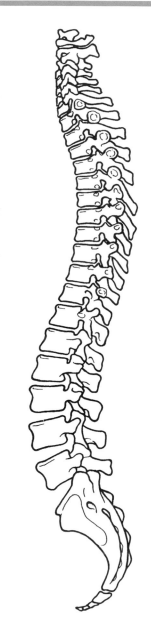

Fig. 20.2 Curves in the spine

Synovial joints

Most of the body's joints are synovial. The space between the bones is filled with synovial fluid and is often capable of a wide range of movement. The synovial fluid in these joints allows frictionless movement between articulating bones. There are several types of synovial joints.

i) Ball and socket joint, e.g. hip and shoulder.

ii) Gliding joint, e.g. carpal (wrist) and tarsal (foot) joints.

iii) Pivot joint, e.g. atlas-axis joint in the cervical vertebrae.

iv) Hinge joint, e.g. elbow and ankle.

v) Condyloid joint, e.g. knee and knuckles.

vi) Saddle joint, e.g. base of the thumb.

3 The vertebral column

The spine consists of seven cervical, twelve thoracic, five lumbar bones, five sacral bones fused to form the sacrum, and four fused vertebrae of the coccyx, forming a nonprotruding 'tail' articulating with the sacrum.

The atlas and axis

The atlas and axis are two special vertebrae at the very top of the skull. They allow rotation of the head.

The cervical vertebrae

The cervical vertebrae are finer and less dense as they only have to support the weight of the skull.

The thoracic vertebrae

The thoracic vertebrae are finer and have less density as they are not weight bearing. Their main function is to support the structure of the rib cage.

The lumbar vertebrae

Lumbar vertebrae are much denser and stronger than the thoracic vertebrae because the whole weight of the body is supported from this section.

The curves in the spine

See Figure 20.2. We have three gentle curves in the spine. The cervical and lumbar sections curve slightly forwards, whilst the thoracic section curves backwards.

Diseases of the spinal column which create exaggerated abnormal curves are: scoliosis, when the

FOOT CHART

FOOT CHART

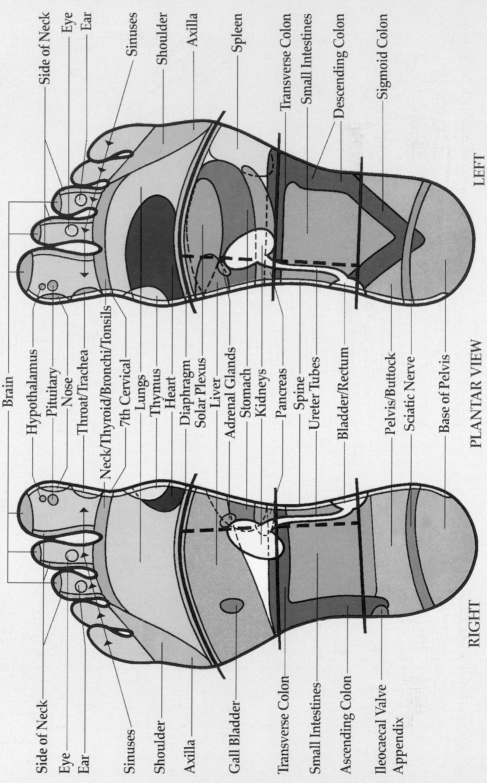

RIGHT

LEFT

PLANTAR VIEW

Brain
Hypothalamus
Pituitary
Nose
Throat/Trachea
Neck/Thyroid/Bronchi/Tonsils
7th Cervical
Lungs
Thymus
Heart
Diaphragm
Solar Plexus
Liver
Adrenal Glands
Stomach
Kidneys
Pancreas
Spine
Ureter Tubes
Bladder/Rectum
Pelvis/Buttock
Sciatic Nerve
Base of Pelvis

Side of Neck
Eye
Ear
Sinuses
Shoulder
Axilla
Spleen
Transverse Colon
Small Intestines
Descending Colon
Sigmoid Colon

Side of Neck
Eye
Ear
Sinuses
Shoulder
Axilla
Gall Bladder
Transverse Colon
Small Intestines
Ascending Colon
Ileocaecal Valve
Appendix

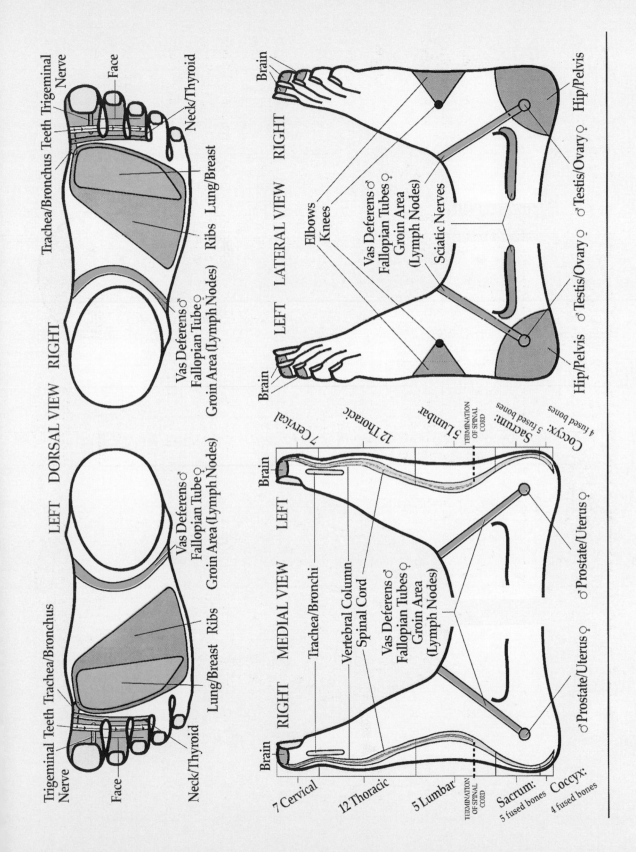

Trachea/Bronchus Teeth Trigeminal Nerve
Face
Neck/Thyroid
Ribs Lung/Breast
Vas Deferens♂ Fallopian Tube♀ Groin Area (Lymph Nodes)

RIGHT DORSAL VIEW LEFT

Trigeminal Teeth Trachea/Bronchus Nerve
Face
Neck/Thyroid
Lung/Breast Ribs
Vas Deferens♂ Fallopian Tube♀ Groin Area (Lymph Nodes)

Brain
RIGHT LATERAL VIEW LEFT
Brain

Elbows
Knees
Vas Deferens♂ Fallopian Tubes♀ Groin Area (Lymph Nodes)
Sciatic Nerves

Hip/Pelvis
♂Testis/Ovary♀
♂Testis/Ovary♀ Hip/Pelvis

7 Cervical
12 Thoracic
5 Lumbar
TERMINATION OF SPINAL CORD
Sacrum: 5 fused bones
Coccyx: 4 fused bones

Brain
LEFT MEDIAL VIEW RIGHT
Brain

Trachea/Bronchi
Vertebral Column Spinal Cord
Vas Deferens♂ Fallopian Tubes♀ Groin Area (Lymph Nodes)

♂Prostate/Uterus♀
♂Prostate/Uterus♀

7 Cervical
12 Thoracic
5 Lumbar
TERMINATION OF SPINAL CORD
Sacrum: 5 fused bones
Coccyx: 4 fused bones

spine resembles an S shape; lordosis, when the lumbar spine bends forwards causing your low abdominal area to bulge forwards and kyphosis, when there is a hump appearance in the thoracic spine.

4 Discs

The main joints between the vertebrae of the spine are cartilaginous joints and are slightly mobile. The vertebral surface is covered with hyaline cartilage and the intervening space is filled with a thick ring of fibrocartilage with a centre of soft, almost gelatinous tissue. The joints are held together by the anterior and posterior longitudinal ligaments and muscles.

The spinal vertebrae also have joints between their other articulating surfaces on the neural arches and with the ribs in the thoracic region. These have a synovial membrane and are surrounded by ligaments. This allows a much greater degree of movement.

The joints between the atlas and occiput and between the atlas and axis do not have discs but rely on synovial membranes to give movement. The intervertebral discs act as shock absorbers. The movement between the individual vertebrae, with the exception of the axis and atlas is small, but the overall combining effect is considerable.

Most of the flexion and extension is in the cervical and lumbar regions; bending to the side is principally in the lumbar area.

The intervertebral discs tend to wear through the years and can eventually become very thin. The statement which is common on results from X-rays – 'narrowing of the disc space' – means just that. This explains why old people become shorter as they get older and deterioration of the joints occurs.

We are also a little taller in the morning and become shorter as the day proceeds. As we lay in bed our muscles and ligaments are able to be stretched out, consequently we are taller. As we stand, sit and walk during the day our spines compress and we become shorter.

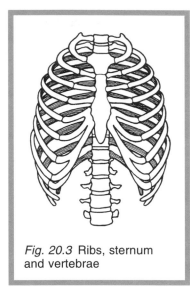

Fig. 20.3 Ribs, sternum and vertebrae

5 The thorax

See Figure 20.3. The thorax consists of twelve pairs of ribs articulating with the thoracic vertebrae; seven pairs attached directly to the sternum by costal cartilage; three pairs of false ribs attached to the sternum by a common bar of cartilage to the rib above and two pairs of floating ribs not connected to the sternum.

Conditions benefiting from reflexology – how reflexology can help

The cartilage discs that separate one vertebrae from another have a hard outer covering and a jelly like centre. Pressure or injury may rupture the outer layer causing pressing on spinal root nerves and this is the main cause for intense back pain and disability. We often hear this condition referred to as a 'slipped disc'.

There are obviously limitations in what we can achieve in degenerative conditions of the spine in the elderly; but generally reflexology can offer some reduction in pain and stiffness, reduce inflammation, and give the patient a better quality of life.

The reflex points to the spine are absolutely vital in the treatment of reflexology. Stimulation of the reflexes helps relax tense muscles and ligaments restoring lightness and mobility to the skeleton.

Back conditions are all too common today and the usual medical approach for back pain is normally pain-killing and anti-inflammatory medications, and in many instances complete bed rest.

Physiotherapy is often advised, and sometimes helps the condition. However reflexology can give immense relief to spinal conditions.

A variety of discomforts from lumbago, to sciatica and whiplash injuries which affect both the neck and lumbar regions have all responded admirably to reflexology treatments. In fact, I would say that reflexologists treat more patients with back conditions that any other form of health problem.

Remember the central nervous system and the area to the vertebral column in the spine share exactly the same reflex points within the foot, as the spinal cord

> Reflexology can give immense relief to spinal conditions

actually extends from the foramen magnum, a hole in the base of the skull, to the second lumbar vertebrae.

Back conditions are on the increase and this is due mainly to the fact that man has grown so much in a very short period of time. It was not very long ago when a man of average height could walk quite freely through the door of a small country cottage. It is hardly possible for anybody to be able to walk through these low doorways to-day. Our teenagers are growing to be quite tall due in the main to the decrease in infant disease. Rickets and rheumatic fever are, thankfully, a thing of the past and the great improvement in nutrition and the care and welfare of infants is quite considerable, particularly in the western world.

Generally speaking, the taller you are the more likely you will be to suffer from back conditions, simply because the spine has more to support.

A person with a shorter, fatter body has less trouble with back troubles, plus the fact that when there is more body fat, there is a higher oestrogen content – oestrogen does help the mobility of our joints and retains a good calcium level in bone. The disadvantage is that high oestrogen levels, increase the likelihood of cancer.

Many of the pains in our knees are the result of lumbar spinal problems and it is interesting to find on X-ray that nothing is wrong with the knee joint and that the problem is arising from compression or wear and tear in the lumbar spine

The feet never lie – reflexology finds the source of the trouble

The feet never lie. When there is a sensitivity in reflex points in the feet there is always a corresponding problem in the physical body.

We are also able to treat frozen shoulders, most successfully, and reflexology helps with freeing tension and pain in cases of arthritis.

Tennis elbow, chronic neck inflammations, cases of arthritis of the cervical spine, sciatica or the damage caused by a whiplash injury, are all common conditions and can be eased with reflexology treatments.

Although we need to treat the patient for many weeks, we do achieve good results in treating sciatic pain.

Areas to work to help the muscular system

The muscular system is distributed throughout the body and we do not need to isolate on the feet, specific areas to help the muscular system as these are worked out when we work with reflexology on the entire body. Working on Zone 1 – the brain and spinal column would assist stimulation of muscles through excitation of nerves.

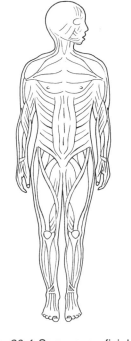

Fig. 20.4 Some superficial muscles of the body

THE MUSCULAR SYSTEM

All body movements such as walking, running, talking, eating food and the circulation of blood and lymph depend on the action of muscles.

Muscle tissue is composed of cells specialized to contract and are normally referred to as muscle fibres rather than cells. Muscle fibres are arranged in layers surrounded by connective tissue.

There are three types of muscle in the body, namely, skeletal muscle, cardiac muscle and smooth muscle.

Skeletal muscle fibres

These have a striated appearance and are voluntary muscles. They are attached to bones and when they contract they pull on bones and move parts of the body.

Smooth muscle fibres

These are not striated, control is involuntary and occurs in the walls of the digestive tract, blood vessels, lymph vessels, uterus and other internal organs.

Cardiac muscle and smooth muscle are discussed in Chapters 6, 10, 12 and 24. Here we will focus on skeletal muscle, the voluntary muscle attached to bone.

There are approximately 600 skeletal muscles in the body. Each skeletal muscle is an organ which produces movement by contraction controlled by motor nerves. Muscle contraction requires energy and the immediate source comes from the energy storage molecule ATP (adenosine triphosphate).

Muscle tone is a state of partial contraction of a skeletal muscle. Even when we are not moving, our muscles remain slightly contracted, ready for action. When the motor nerve to a muscle is severed the muscle becomes limp.

Skeletal muscles are attached to bones by tendons and movements are produced when muscles contract, pulling on tendons which in turn pull on bones. Movements are brought about by groups of muscles working together. The agonists are muscles which produce a particular action and the antagonists are muscles which cause the opposite action.

CHAPTER 21 Practical procedures for working the skeletal and muscular systems

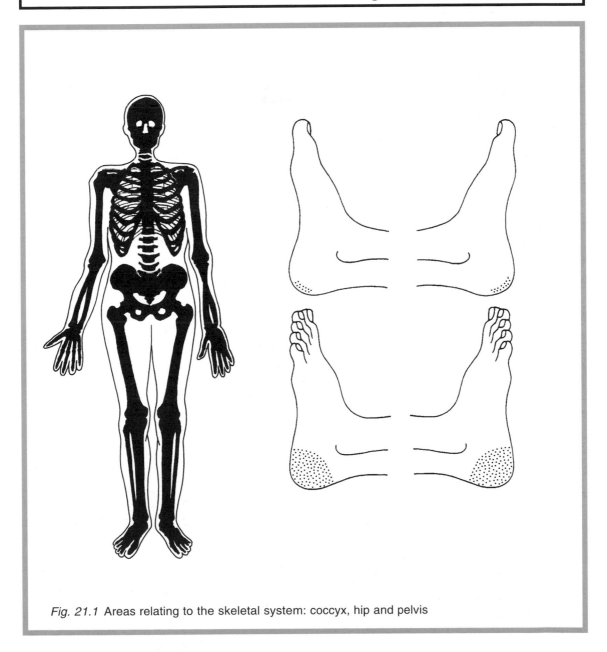

Fig. 21.1 Areas relating to the skeletal system: coccyx, hip and pelvis

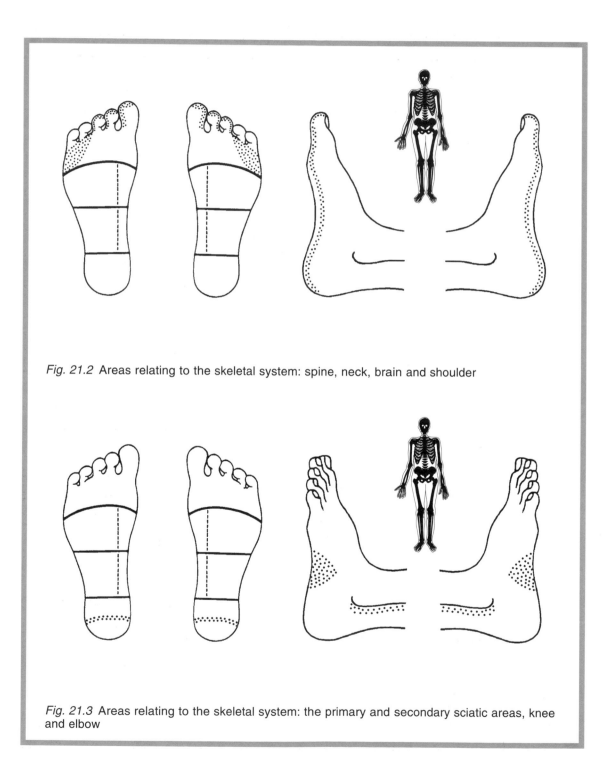

Fig. 21.2 Areas relating to the skeletal system: spine, neck, brain and shoulder

Fig. 21.3 Areas relating to the skeletal system: the primary and secondary sciatic areas, knee and elbow

1 The vertebral column: Coccyx Zone 1 Hip/pelvis Zone 5 – *right foot*

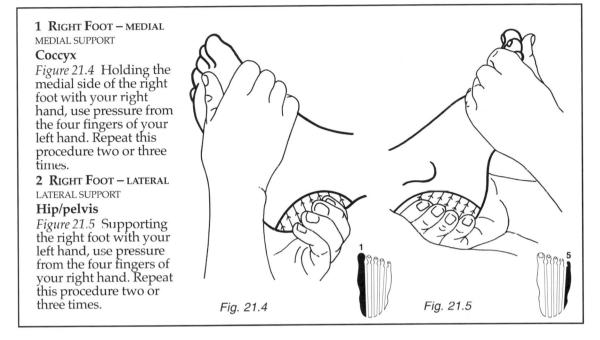

1 RIGHT FOOT – MEDIAL
MEDIAL SUPPORT
Coccyx
Figure 21.4 Holding the medial side of the right foot with your right hand, use pressure from the four fingers of your left hand. Repeat this procedure two or three times.

2 RIGHT FOOT – LATERAL
LATERAL SUPPORT
Hip/pelvis
Figure 21.5 Supporting the right foot with your left hand, use pressure from the four fingers of your right hand. Repeat this procedure two or three times.

Fig. 21.4   Fig. 21.5

2 The vertebral column – Zone 1 Cervical spine Zone 1 – *right foot*

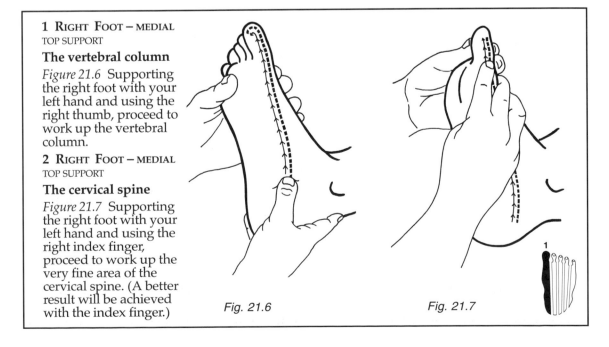

1 RIGHT FOOT – MEDIAL
TOP SUPPORT

The vertebral column

Figure 21.6 Supporting the right foot with your left hand and using the right thumb, proceed to work up the vertebral column.

2 RIGHT FOOT – MEDIAL
TOP SUPPORT

The cervical spine

Figure 21.7 Supporting the right foot with your left hand and using the right index finger, proceed to work up the very fine area of the cervical spine. (A better result will be achieved with the index finger.)

Fig. 21.6   Fig. 21.7

3 The vertebral column – Zone 1 **Chronic neck** Zones 1 2 3 – *right foot*

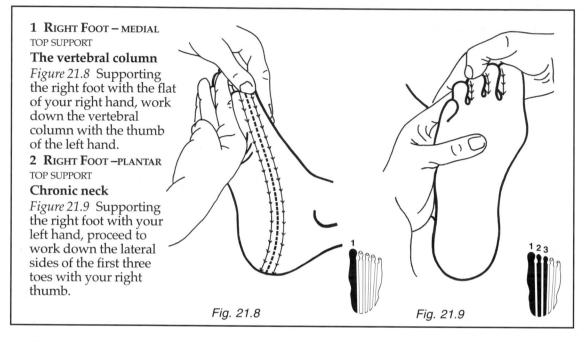

1 RIGHT FOOT – MEDIAL
TOP SUPPORT
The vertebral column
Figure 21.8 Supporting the right foot with the flat of your right hand, work down the vertebral column with the thumb of the left hand.

2 RIGHT FOOT –PLANTAR
TOP SUPPORT
Chronic neck
Figure 21.9 Supporting the right foot with your left hand, proceed to work down the lateral sides of the first three toes with your right thumb.

Fig. 21.8   Fig. 21.9

4 The shoulder area – *right foot* Zones 4 5

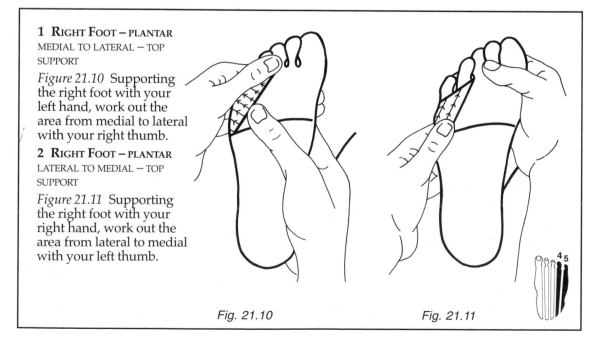

1 RIGHT FOOT – PLANTAR
MEDIAL TO LATERAL – TOP SUPPORT

Figure 21.10 Supporting the right foot with your left hand, work out the area from medial to lateral with your right thumb.

2 RIGHT FOOT – PLANTAR
LATERAL TO MEDIAL – TOP SUPPORT

Figure 21.11 Supporting the right foot with your right hand, work out the area from lateral to medial with your left thumb.

Fig. 21.10   Fig. 21.11

5 The knee/elbow area – *right foot* Zone 5

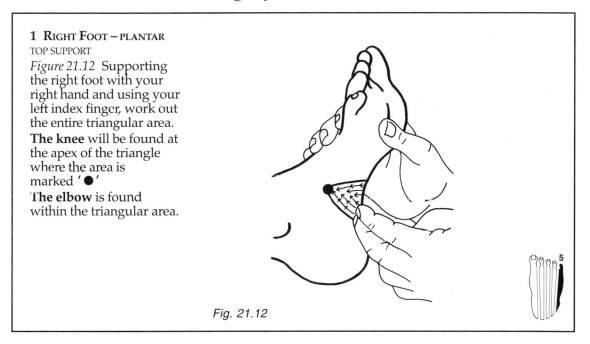

1 RIGHT FOOT – PLANTAR
TOP SUPPORT
Figure 21.12 Supporting the right foot with your right hand and using your left index finger, work out the entire triangular area.

The knee will be found at the apex of the triangle where the area is marked '●'

The elbow is found within the triangular area.

Fig. 21.12

6 The sciatic areas: **Primary** Zone 5 **Secondary** Zones 1 2 3 4 5 – *right foot*

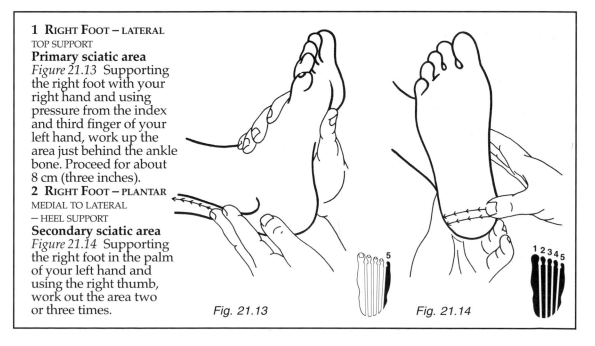

1 RIGHT FOOT – LATERAL
TOP SUPPORT
Primary sciatic area
Figure 21.13 Supporting the right foot with your right hand and using pressure from the index and third finger of your left hand, work up the area just behind the ankle bone. Proceed for about 8 cm (three inches).

2 RIGHT FOOT – PLANTAR
MEDIAL TO LATERAL
– HEEL SUPPORT
Secondary sciatic area
Figure 21.14 Supporting the right foot in the palm of your left hand and using the right thumb, work out the area two or three times.

Fig. 21.13   *Fig. 21.14*

7 The vertebral column: Coccyx Zone 1 Hip/pelvis Zone 5 – *left foot*

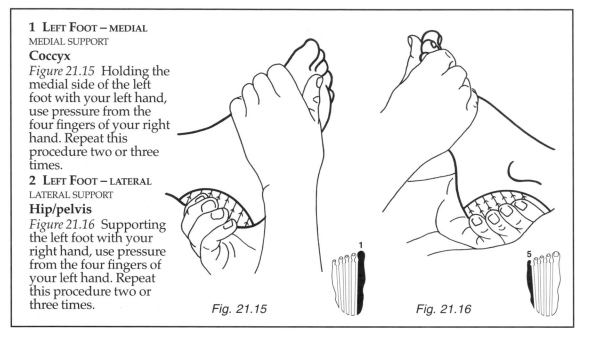

1 LEFT FOOT – MEDIAL
MEDIAL SUPPORT

Coccyx

Figure 21.15 Holding the medial side of the left foot with your left hand, use pressure from the four fingers of your right hand. Repeat this procedure two or three times.

2 LEFT FOOT – LATERAL
LATERAL SUPPORT

Hip/pelvis

Figure 21.16 Supporting the left foot with your right hand, use pressure from the four fingers of your left hand. Repeat this procedure two or three times.

Fig. 21.15   *Fig. 21.16*

8 The vertebral column – Zone 1 Cervical spine Zone 1 – *left foot*

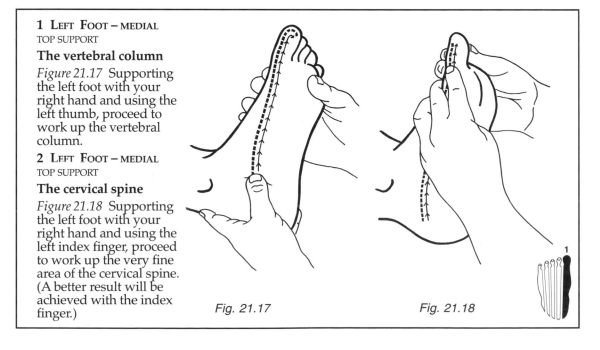

1 LEFT FOOT – MEDIAL
TOP SUPPORT

The vertebral column

Figure 21.17 Supporting the left foot with your right hand and using the left thumb, proceed to work up the vertebral column.

2 LEFT FOOT – MEDIAL
TOP SUPPORT

The cervical spine

Figure 21.18 Supporting the left foot with your right hand and using the left index finger, proceed to work up the very fine area of the cervical spine. (A better result will be achieved with the index finger.)

Fig. 21.17   *Fig. 21.18*

9 The vertebral column – Zone 1 **Chronic neck** Zones 1 2 3 – *left foot*

1 LEFT FOOT – MEDIAL
TOP SUPPORT
The vertebral column
Figure 21.19 Supporting the left foot with the flat of your left hand, work down the vertebral column with the thumb of the right hand.

2 LEFT FOOT – PLANTAR
TOP SUPPORT
Chronic neck
Figure 21.20 Supporting the left foot with your right hand, proceed to work down the lateral sides of the first three toes with your left thumb.

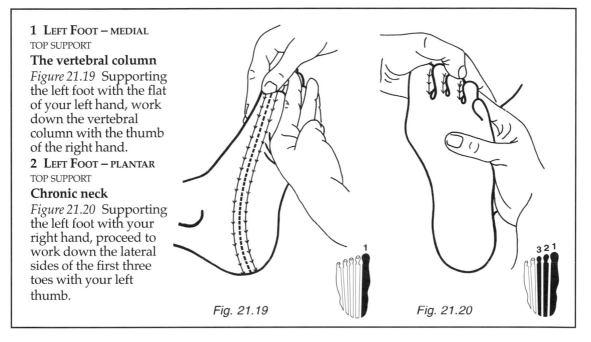

Fig. 21.19   Fig. 21.20

10 The shoulder area – *left foot* Zones 4 5

1 LEFT FOOT – PLANTAR
MEDIAL TO LATERAL
– TOP SUPPORT

Figure 21.21 Supporting the left foot with your right hand, work out the area from medial to lateral with your left thumb.

2 LEFT FOOT – PLANTAR
LATERAL TO MEDIAL
– TOP SUPPORT

Figure 21.22 Supporting the left foot with your left hand, work out the area from lateral to medial with your right thumb.

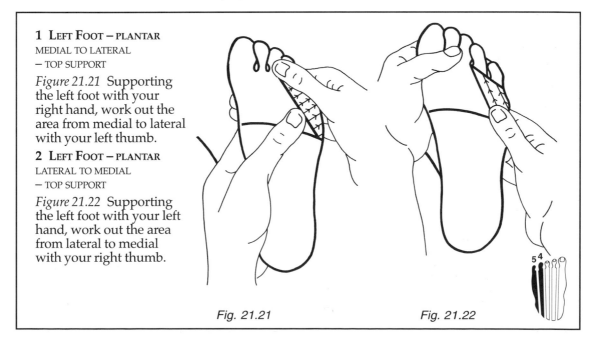

Fig. 21.21   Fig. 21.22

11 The knee/elbow area – *left foot* Zone 5

1 LEFT FOOT – PLANTAR
TOP SUPPORT
Figure 21.23 Supporting the left foot with your left hand and using your right index finger, work out the entire triangular area.

The knee will be found at the apex of the triangle where the area is marked '●'

The elbow is found within the triangular area.

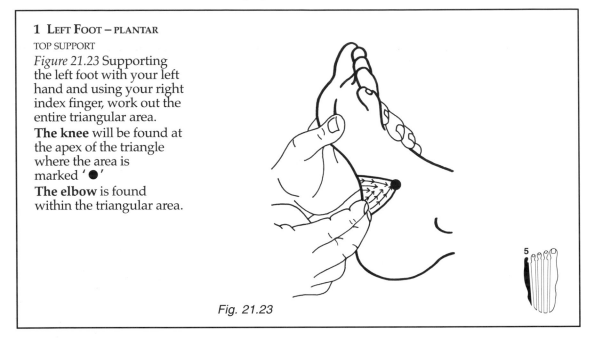

Fig. 21.23

12 The sciatic areas: Primary Zone 5 Secondary Zones 1 2 3 4 5 – *left foot*

1 LEFT FOOT – LATERAL
TOP SUPPORT
Primary sciatic area
Figure 21.24 Supporting the left foot with your left hand and using pressure from the index and third finger of your right hand, work up the area just behind the ankle bone. Proceed for about 8 cm (three inches).

2 LEFT FOOT – PLANTAR
MEDIAL TO LATERAL
– HEEL SUPPORT
Secondary sciatic area
Figure 21.25 Supporting the left foot in the palm of your right hand and using the left thumb, work out the area two or three times.

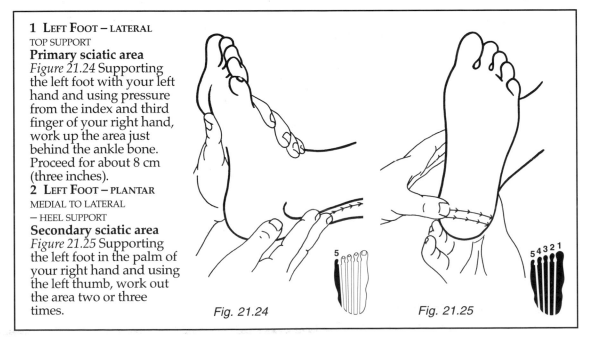

Fig. 21.24

Fig. 21.25

CHAPTER **22** The urinary system

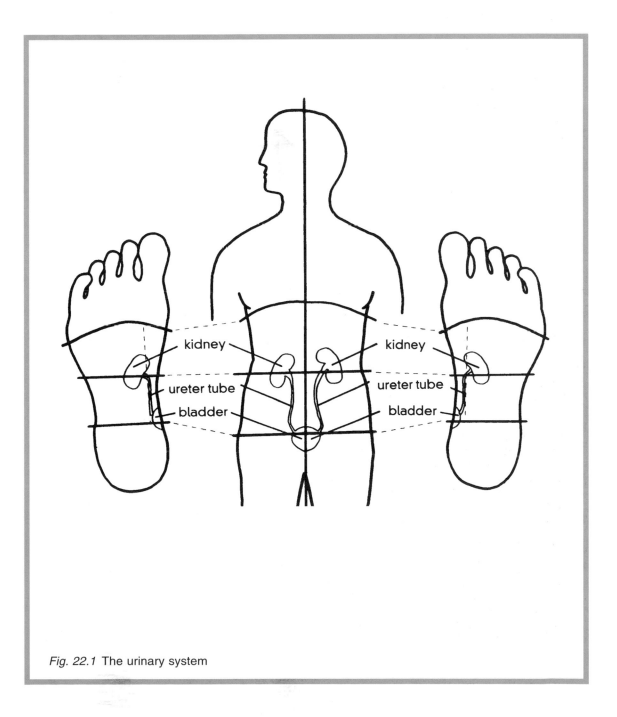

Fig. 22.1 The urinary system

THE URINARY SYSTEM

The urinary system comprises two kidneys, two ureter tubes and a bladder.

1 The kidneys

See Fig. 22.2. The kidneys are a pair of organs which remove metabolic waste. If permitted to accumulate, these wastes could reach toxic concentrations. The kidneys are bean shaped organs, encapsulated in fat. They lie behind the stomach and face inwards towards the spine and together the kidneys are the same size as their owner's heart.

The cortex and medulla

The cortex and medulla contain tiny blood filtration units called nephrons. A single kidney has more than a million nephrons. Urine, the waste product of filtration collects in the kidney's pelvis. Blood for processing enters the medulla from the renal artery, which branches directly from the aorta, the main artery in the body.

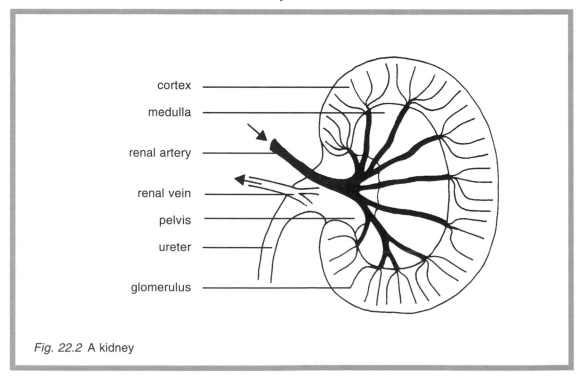

Fig. 22.2 A kidney

Glomeruli

Inside the cortex and medulla the artery splits into tiny coiled blood vessels. Each coiled blood vessel is called a glomerulus. Almost completely surrounding each lies a sac the size of a pin head called the Bowman's capsule. The filtered liquid then continues through a tubule surrounded by capillaries.

These tiny blood vessels reabsorb into the blood most of the water and useful chemicals such as amino acids and glucose. The treated blood then leaves the kidney via the renal vein.

Urine

Meanwhile wastes remaining in the convoluted tubule flow on via a collecting tube to the kidney's pelvis. These wastes now form urine, an amber liquid largely made of water, nitrogen wastes mainly urea, inorganic salts and other substances. From the kidney's pelvis urine leaves the kidney through a tube known as the ureter. The urinary bladder stores urine before it leaves the body. One pair of kidneys can process 180 litres (45 gallons) of blood a day. Urine output drops in sleep or during perspiration and rises after more liquid than usual has been drunk.

2 The ureters

The two ureters connect the bladder to the kidneys. A broader tube, the urethra opens from the bottom of the bladder. A ring of muscles called the urethral sphincter normally keeps this outlet closed.

3 The bladder

The urinary bladder lying in the pelvis, behind the pubic bone, is a temporary storage sac for urine. The lining of the bladder is in folds which permits stretching. An empty bladder is flat, a full bladder can hold about a pint of urine. Urine drips into the bladder through the ureter tubes and the bladder walls relax as it fills. When the bladder holds about a cup full of urine, nerves start sending signals to the brain to urinate. Urination occurs when the external urethral sphincter muscle relaxes and the bladder wall contracts forcing urine through the urethra.

The importance of water

Water is an essential constituent of all life, every living thing depends on water for its survival and it accounts for around 60 per cent of an adult's body weight.

Different tissues hold different amounts of water, fat holds little moisture, while the blood, muscles and skin have high concentrations. Water transports hormones and nutrients around the body which helps to dilute toxic substances and absorb waste products.

To remain healthy we really do need to drink about 2 litres (nearly half a gallon) of fluid daily: few people do.

We are losing bodily fluids constantly in exhaled air and perspiration and also the fluid content which is passed when we open our bowels.

The kidneys need sufficient fluid to produce urine which keeps the body's chemistry in balance.

How reflexology can help in the treatment of urinary conditions

A female bladder is situated in the pelvis below the uterus hence the fact that women in pregnancy have the frequent desire to urinate. In the male, the urethra is long and passes through the prostate gland and the penis. In the female the urethra is short and opens to the outside just above the vagina. Bladder infections are more common in females than males because the long male urethra is a barrier to bacterial invasion.

The most common inflammatory state of the bladder is called cystitis, which is caused by bacteria invading the delicate membranes of the bladder causing pain, frequent urination and a feeling of being generally unwell.

The male bladder has a prostate gland encircling the urethra, which is at the base, and as men grow older its enlargement may compress the urethra causing problems with frequency of urination. Cancer of the prostate is a common disorder in men over 50 years.

The male urethra is about 20 cm (8 in) long. Its role is to transport semen and urine from the body.

The consistency and smell of urine varies from what we eat and drink. When you drink a large amount of water, you kidneys produce a large volume of urine which is a light straw colour. When you drink too little water, only a small amount of urine is produced and is a dark brown colour.

Medical tests are conducted on urine which enables various malfunctions in the body to be picked up: toxaemia in pregnancy is but one condition which usually results in protein being present in the urine. This raises alarm as it means that the kidneys are finding the pregnancy just a little too stressful – eliminating waste products for two beings instead of one. Protein in the urine, plus a rise in blood pressure together with puffy ankles and fingers would certainly need immediate attention from a specialist in deciding whether bed rest would improve the situation, or whether the mother and baby would both benefit from an early delivery.

Urinary incontinence is the tendency to involuntary leakage of urine. It can happen when you suddenly cough or sneeze, or pick up a heavy object. It occurs more in women than in men mainly because women often have a weakness in their pelvic floor muscles if they have had children, or a difficult birth which resulted in a forceps delivery.

Incontinence is especially common in elderly people and often accompanies senile dementia. Damage to the spinal cord as the result of an accident in the lumbar spinal area is yet another cause of incontinence

Reflexology has proved to be very successful in relieving the conditions mentioned above.

Long term diabetes can lead to complications in the kidney function and may progress to kidney failure.

Kidney stones are common, more frequent in males than females. Certain concentrated substances in the urine may produce kidney stones and these may form in the urine collecting part of the kidneys or the ureter tubes. Both these conditions are extremely painful. In fact renal pain has been said to be the most excruciating pain that one can suffer.

As the kidneys face inwards towards the spine in the lumbar region, kidney pain can often be confused with back pain and therefore sometimes 'put up with' for a long period of time before consulting with a doctor – X-rays will reveal that there are stones in the kidney.

Nephritis, which is inflammation of the small nephrons in the kidney, is yet another condition which has been most successfully treated with reflexology.

High blood pressure has close associations with the kidneys. Patients suffering from chronic hypertension often find that the kidney function can eventually become impaired. The increased pressure being forced through the kidney tubules often causes a collapse of these delicate nephrons and a less efficient function of the filtering system, so it is common to find that those suffering from high blood pressure will have very sensitive reflexes in the kidney areas.

By taking the stress off the kidneys we are able in turn to improve the kidney function which has an effect on lowering the blood pressure.

Be sure to work out the areas connected to the pelvic hip and coccyx area and also the lumbar spine when treating bladder and kidney problems.

I feel that by stimulating the whole pelvic cavity we are able to break down a lot of stress and tension and help rid the body of its impurities.

CHAPTER 23 Practical procedures for working the urinary system

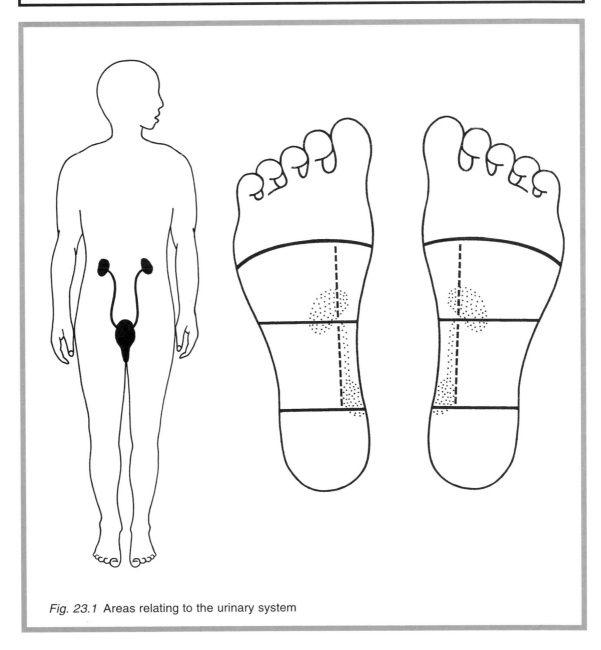

Fig. 23.1 Areas relating to the urinary system

1 **The bladder/ureter tube** – Zones 1 2 **The kidney** Zone 2 – *right foot*

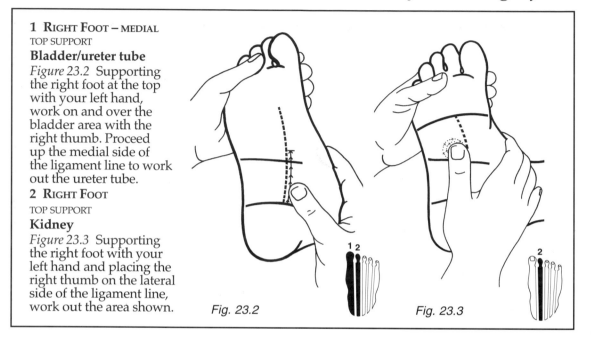

1 RIGHT FOOT – MEDIAL
TOP SUPPORT
Bladder/ureter tube
Figure 23.2 Supporting the right foot at the top with your left hand, work on and over the bladder area with the right thumb. Proceed up the medial side of the ligament line to work out the ureter tube.

2 RIGHT FOOT
TOP SUPPORT
Kidney
Figure 23.3 Supporting the right foot with your left hand and placing the right thumb on the lateral side of the ligament line, work out the area shown.

Fig. 23.2

Fig. 23.3

2 **The bladder/ureter tube** – Zones 1 2 **The kidney** Zone 2 – *left foot*

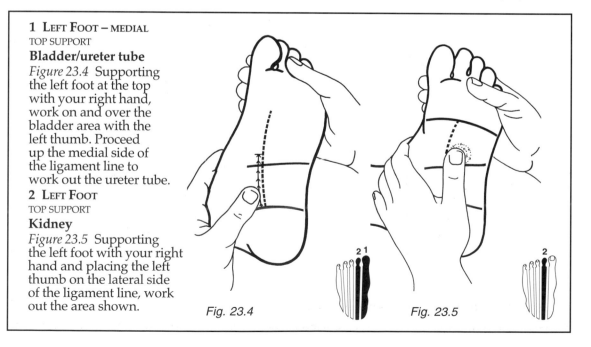

1 LEFT FOOT – MEDIAL
TOP SUPPORT
Bladder/ureter tube
Figure 23.4 Supporting the left foot at the top with your right hand, work on and over the bladder area with the left thumb. Proceed up the medial side of the ligament line to work out the ureter tube.

2 LEFT FOOT
TOP SUPPORT
Kidney
Figure 23.5 Supporting the left foot with your right hand and placing the left thumb on the lateral side of the ligament line, work out the area shown.

Fig. 23.4

Fig. 23.5

CHAPTER **24** The reproductive system

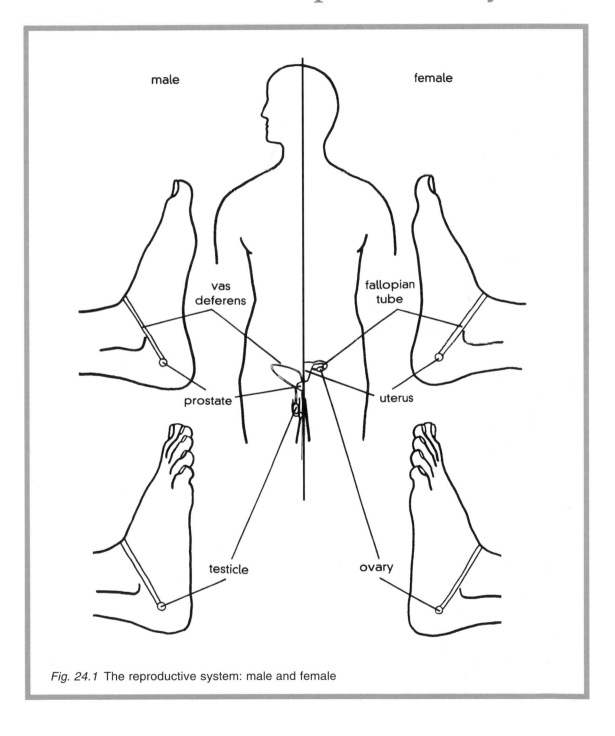

Fig. 24.1 The reproductive system: male and female

THE REPRODUCTIVE SYSTEM

1 The female reproductive organs

See Figure 24.2. The essential sex glands in the woman are two ovaries which produce ova to maintain the act of procreation. Apart from the importance of the ovaries, the female reproductive system has to provide nutrition to the fertilised ovum and protect it until the pregnancy ends.

The ovaries and ovulation

Ovaries are small, oblong, pearl-coloured organs that lie just below the fallopian tubes on each side of the uterus.

Ovaries produce eggs: a woman has the greatest number of eggs in her ovaries that she will ever have – about 20 million – when she is a 20 week foetus inside her mother's womb. Our biological time clock for reproduction begins ticking before we are even born.

Our ovaries produce eggs about once a month, from about the age of 13 or 14 onwards. Maturation is controlled by FSH from the pituitary gland. Cells of the follicles in the ovaries secrete oestrogen. Ovulation causes a small cyst to erupt each month and this eruption releases a watery fluid, encouraging the ova to be propelled out of the ovary. This surrounding fluid is known as liquor folliculi.

The fallopian tubes, 12 cm long with their moving finger-like projections called fimbriae, draw the ovum into the tube. Peristaltic contractions in the muscular wall and the cilia help move the ovum toward the uterus.

LH from the pituitary gland stimulates the development of the corpus luteum which temporarily secretes progesterone and oestrogen. These hormones stimulate the uterus to prepare for a possible pregnancy.

At the time of ovulation many women get ovulation pain. It is interesting to find that you can pick up, via the feet, which ovary is releasing the ova.

If ovulation is occurring on the right side you will find quite a sensitive reaction when you apply pressure on the right foot. If ovulation occurs on the left side a sensitive reaction will be found on the left foot. Reflexology picks up the sensitivity in the ovary, as it does in any other part of the body that is inflamed, congested or tense.

Ovaries decrease in size when the reproductive years are over, but ovarian function still produces hormones which help our general health.

Our ovaries should be respected and considered as valuable organs which can go on maintaining hormonal output throughout our life.

In many Taoist cultures the ovaries are thought to contain the life force that produces sexual energy.

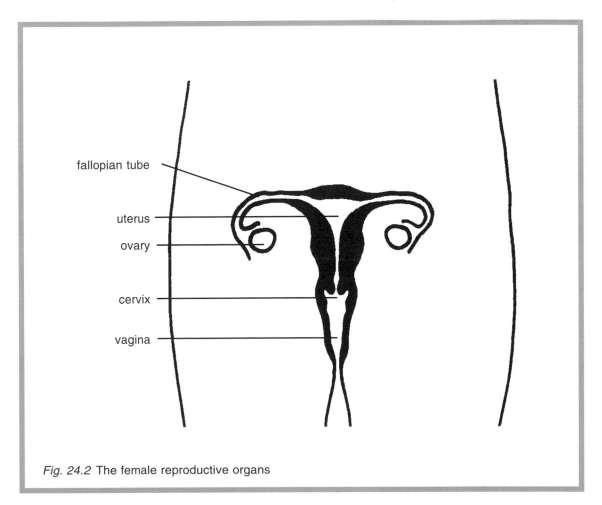

Fig. 24.2 The female reproductive organs

The vagina

At the entrance to the vagina are a pair of lip like folds – the larger and thicker being the labia majora, and the smaller and inner being the labia minora.

They lie on either side of the vaginal entrance and join in the front, blending into the padded area of the mons pubis. At the front they enclose the exit of the urethra just behind the small projection of tissue, the clitoris, which is comparable to the penis.

Behind these structures is the vagina, a 10–15cm elastic tube, lined with moist epithelium.

Unlike the male urinary system that of the female is separate from the reproductive system. The bladder empties into the urethra which opens in front of the vagina.

Vagina comes from the Latin 'vaina', meaning 'sheath for a sword'.

In prehistoric societies vulvas and pubic triangles were frequently drawn or inscribed on cave walls to symbolise a sacred place, a gateway to life.

The uterus

At the top of the vagina the uterus is held in place by muscles and four strong fibrous ligaments of the pelvic floor and to the side of the pelvis by pairs of round and suspensory ligaments running in folds of peritoneum.

The uterus is a small pear shaped organ covered with peritoneum with a thick wall of interweaving muscle fibres and lined with special endometrial cells. It is situated behind the bladder and in front of the rectum.

The cervix of the uterus is a thick fibrous muscular structure opening into the vagina and lined with special cells that form a plug of mucus. Uterine muscles are always contracting and relaxing slightly.

The umbilical cord

Some native American tribes considered the umbilical cord as a cord of reverence not as a waste product to be discarded at delivery. This long, thin, spiral sinue that is left after birth is a powerful link reflecting the unity and protection that the child had with its mother.

The native Americans wrapped the cord around a stone and laid it to dry in the sun. When completely dried they stored the cord in a container, keeping a record of the child's day, date and time of birth.

The umbilical cord was kept until the child was taught to ride his or her first pony when it was braided into the pony's mane, believing that this mother / child link would still be there, offering protection.

Fertilization

Fertilization takes place high in the fallopian tube when the head of the sperm penetrates the female ovum's outer layer. The female cell is the largest in the human body although it is no larger than the full stop at the end of this paragraph.

The sperm sheds its tail and body while the head, which contains all the genetic material, moves towards the ovum's nucleus. The sperm is propelled by its long tail. The nuclei of the sperm and ovum each contain 23 chromosomes.

Disorders of the female reproductive system

As with other parts of our body the ovaries can be subjected to various diseases: ovarian cysts, polycystic ovaries which are usually due to a hormonal dysfunction and, at the worst, ovarian cancer, which unfortunately is on the increase.

Many cysts erupt of their own accord and that is that. Some become very large and cause pressure and discomfort on organs in the pelvic cavity; these are then treated medicinally or surgically.

Many patients coming for reflexology treatments for ovarian cysts have found that within weeks, the discomfort subsides and the cyst disappears, so it is well worth trying reflexology before you resort to other measures.

A woman suffering from heavy bleeding or large fibroids may relieve herself of many of these unpleasant symptoms if she changes from a high fat and high protein diet, to a low fat, high fibre and mostly vegetarian diet. The standard British diet is precisely the diet that encourages the risk of the development of fibroids and tumours.

It is so worth while trying reflexology and dietary changes first: surgery can always be used as a last resort instead of a first choice.

2 The male reproductive system

See Figure 24.3. The reproductive system comprises in the male, two testes which hang in the scrotal sac, the seminal vesicle, prostate gland, the epididymis and the penis.

The testes

Testes have two functions: the production of testosterone and spermatozoa. Testosterone responds to the gonadotropic hormones from the pituitary gland and causes development of male secondary sexual characteristics – pubic and facial hair growth, aggressiveness, muscle bulk and deepening of the voice.

The tubules inside the testes produce large quantities of sperm every day which pass into a series of communicating ducts.

The epididymis, a coiled tube, empties into the vas deferens and passes from the scrotum through the inguinal canal. The vas deferens is joined by the duct from the seminal vesicles to become the ejaculatory duct. This duct passes through the prostate and and then opens into the urethra.

The seminal vesicle acts as a storage organ for the mature sperm. Secretions of the seminal vesicles account for about 60 per cent of semen volume.

The prostate gland

The prostate gland lies around the first part of the urethra, at the base of the bladder, and its secretions help maintain sperm activity. Two additional pairs of glands, Cowper's, release a few drops of fluid which neutralizes the acidity of the urethra and lubricates the urethra and penis.

The penis

The penis is the male organ of reproduction. It also has another function which is the excretion of urine from the bladder out of the body.

Disorders of the testes

The most common symptom involving the testicle is a swelling. Most swellings are painless and should be checked. Swellings may be due to a collection of fluid called a hydrocele.

There is another condition involving the scrotum where enlargement of the veins causes a varicosity which creates swelling and tenderness in the scrotal area.

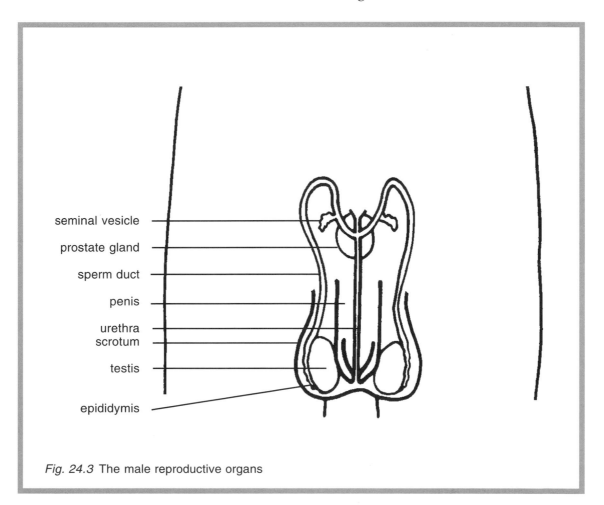

seminal vesicle

prostate gland

sperm duct

penis

urethra
scrotum

testis

epididymis

Fig. 24.3 The male reproductive organs

Disorders of the prostate gland

The prostate gland located at the base of the bladder surrounds the urethra, and its disorders are common in males over 50 years, particularly cancer.

Enlargement of this gland causes a distortion of the urethra, a weakening of the flow of urine and, as the bladder cannot be emptied completely, a tendency for urine infections is common.

CHAPTER 25 Practical procedures for working the reproductive system

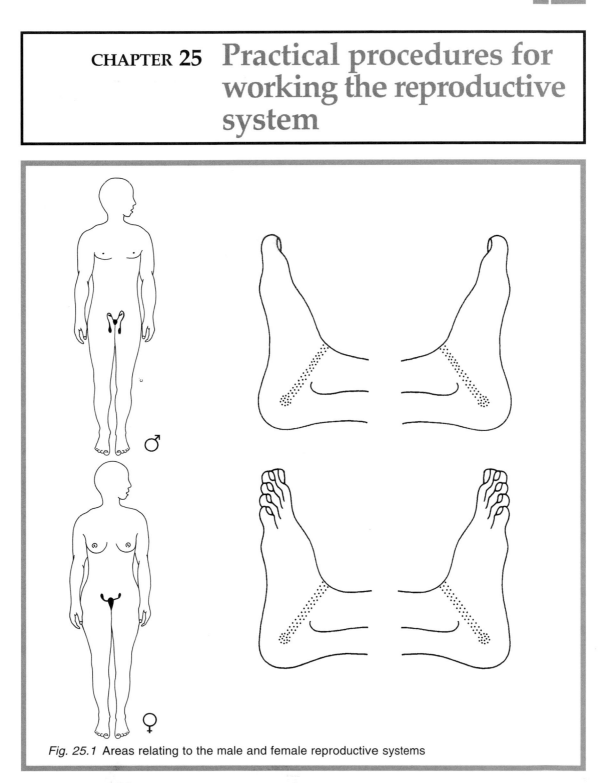

Fig. 25.1 Areas relating to the male and female reproductive systems

1 The uterus/prostate area – *right foot* Zone 1

1 Right Foot – medial
Figure 25.2 These areas are to be found halfway between the ankle bone and the tip of the heel.

2 Right Foot – medial
TOP SUPPORT
Figure 25.3 Supporting the right foot with your left hand and using the right index finger, work in a straight line as identified in *Figure 25.2*. Repeat two or three times.

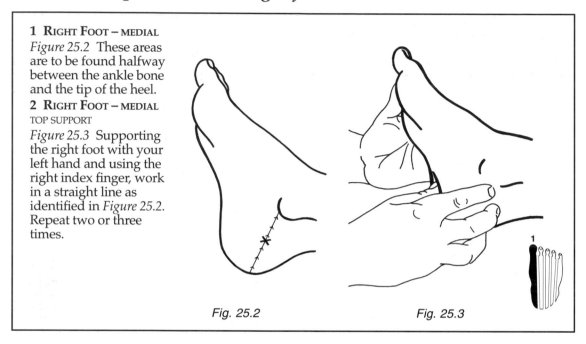

Fig. 25.2   Fig. 25.3

2 The ovary/testis – *right foot* Zone 5

1 Right Foot – lateral
TOP SUPPORT
Figure 25.4 Supporting the right foot with your right hand and using the left index finger, work in a straight line two or three times.

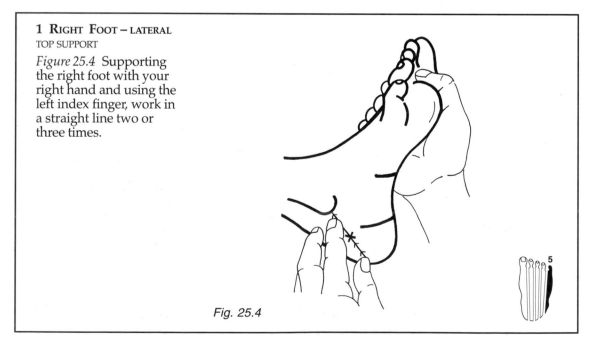

Fig. 25.4

3 Fallopian tubes/Vas deferens – *right foot* Zones 1 2 3 4 5

1 RIGHT FOOT – DORSAL
HEEL SUPPORT
Figure 25.5 Supporting the plantar side of the foot, and pressing in for support with both thumbs, work around the front of the foot with the index and third finger together. Repeat two or three times.

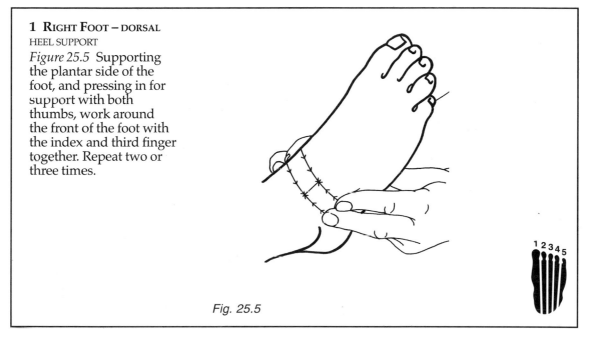

Fig. 25.5

4 The uterus/prostate area – *left foot* Zone 1

1 LEFT FOOT – MEDIAL
Figure 25.6 These areas are to be found halfway between the ankle bone and the tip of the heel.
2 LEFT FOOT – MEDIAL
TOP SUPPORT
Figure 25.7 Supporting the left foot with your right hand and using the left index finger, work in a straight line as identified in *Figure 25.6*. Repeat two or three times.

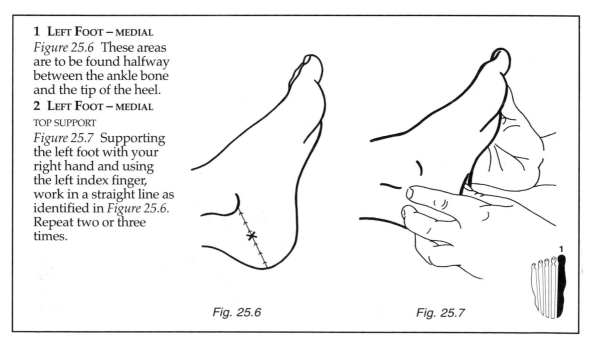

Fig. 25.6

Fig. 25.7

5 The ovary/testis – *left foot* Zone 5

1 Left Foot – LATERAL
TOP SUPPORT

Figure 25.8 Supporting the left foot with your left hand and using the right index finger, work in a straight line two or three times.

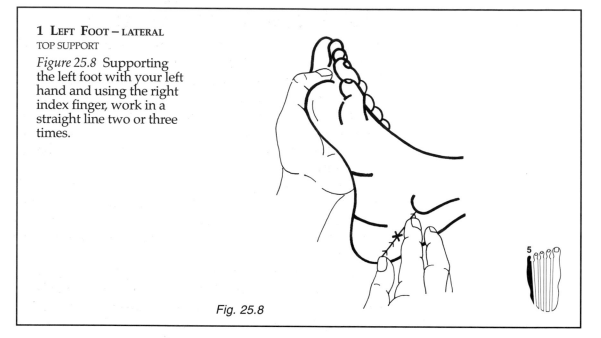

Fig. 25.8

6 Fallopian tubes/Vas deferens – *left foot* Zones 1 2 3 4 5

1 Left Foot – DORSAL
HEEL SUPPORT

Figure 25.9 Supporting the plantar side of the foot, and pressing in for support with both thumbs, work around the front of the foot with the index and third finger together. Repeat two or three times.

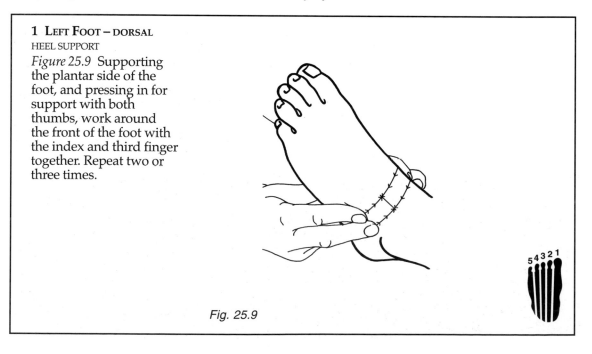

Fig. 25.9

CHAPTER 26 Hand reflexology and the basic hand routine

The benefit of understanding the principle of hand reflexology is that it is easy to work upon your own hands and also, when conditions present themselves in your practice such as with a patient who has a strained ankle, or a diabetic suffering from an ulcerative condition in the foot which makes a foot treatment impossible, you can come to the rescue by giving a hand treatment.

I always show my patients the spinal area in the hand which is quite easy to work upon, and this in turn will stimulate the nerve connections to all parts of the body, as explained in the chapter on The Spinal Connection, Chapter 32.

Apart from helping themselves physically, it is essential that the patient learns to take responsibility for his or her own health problems; this they can do by working daily on their own hands.

The hands are far less sensitive than the feet. Try putting your feet into a very hot bath of water, then place your hands into the same bath. You will be able to sustain far more heat to your hands than you ever can to your feet. Your feet are such sensitive parts of your body: if you stub your toe it can be so terribly painful and can, in fact, make you feel quite sick.

Try wearing tight shoes on a very hot day and walk around the town. The first thing you will do is to kick off your shoes as you get home and stretch your toes, and rotate your ankles. Your feet seem to almost 'smile'

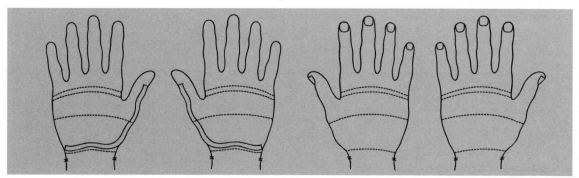

as you do this, and mentally you will begin to relax. Who was it that said 'the pains in her feet were revealed in her face'?

It will be quite easy for you to follow the basic principles of finding the reflex points for appropriate areas by studying the hand chart and seeing that just as reflex points in the feet start with the upper part of the body found in the upper section of the foot and the mid body parts in the mid part of the foot, and the lower areas of the feet reflecting the intestinal, pelvic and urinary system, the reflexes in the hands follow the same pattern.

BASIC HAND REFLEXOLOGY ROUTINE

This is the basic routine to adopt when working on your own hands. These procedures can also be applied in a hand reflexology session, when working on other people's hands and the relaxation techniques explained in the following chapter can only be used on the hands of other people.

1 The lung area – *(a) right hand*

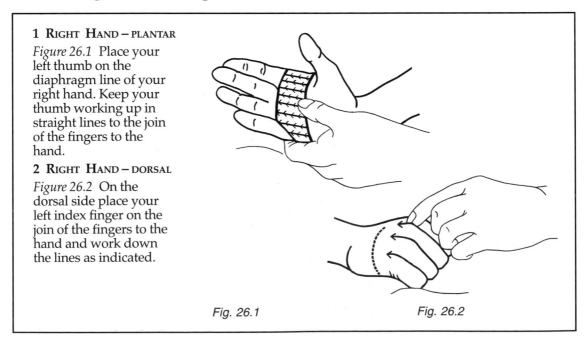

1 RIGHT HAND – PLANTAR

Figure 26.1 Place your left thumb on the diaphragm line of your right hand. Keep your thumb working up in straight lines to the join of the fingers to the hand.

2 RIGHT HAND – DORSAL

Figure 26.2 On the dorsal side place your left index finger on the join of the fingers to the hand and work down the lines as indicated.

Fig. 26.1   Fig. 26.2

2 The lung area – *(b) left hand*

1 LEFT HAND – PLANTAR

Figure 26.3 Place your right thumb on the diaphragm line of your left hand. Keep your thumb working up in straight lines to the join of the fingers to the hand.

2 LEFT HAND – DORSAL

Figure 26.4 On the dorsal side place your right index finger at the join of the fingers to the hand and work down the lines as indicated.

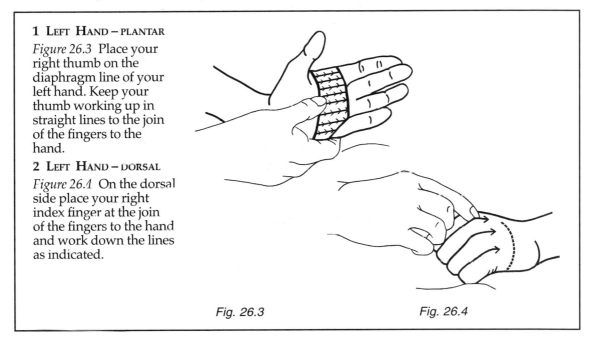

Fig. 26.3   Fig. 26.4

3 The sinuses – *(a) right hand*

1 RIGHT HAND – PLANTAR

Figure 26.5 Commence working on your right hand, and use the left thumb to work out the reflex points to all the fingers. Work in the direction of the arrows as shown.

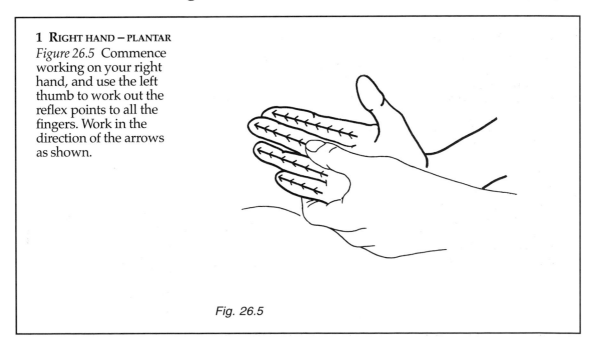

Fig. 26.5

4 The sinuses – *(b) left hand*

1 LEFT HAND – PLANTAR
Figure 26.6 Commence working on your left hand, and use the right thumb to work out the reflex points to all the fingers. Work in the direction of the arrows as shown.

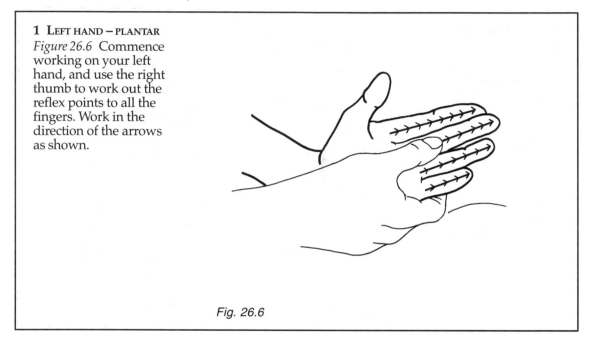

Fig. 26.6

5 The eye and ear – *(a) right hand*

1 RIGHT HAND – PLANTAR
The eye
Figure 26.7 Using your left thumb, apply pressure to the first bend of the index finger of your right hand: use a rotating movement.

2 RIGHT HAND – PLANTAR
The ear
Figure 26.8 Using your left thumb, apply pressure to the first bend of the third finger of your right hand: use a rotating movement.

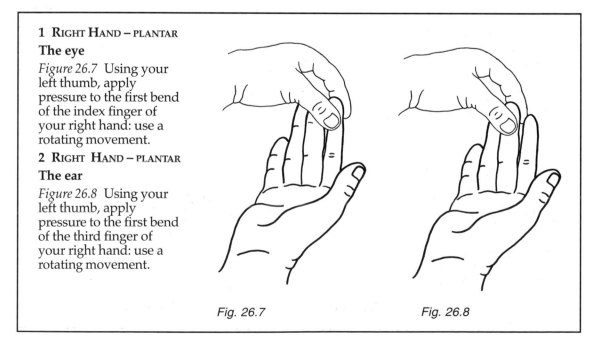

Fig. 26.7   Fig. 26.8

6 The eye and ear – (b) left hand

1 LEFT HAND – PLANTAR

The eye

Figure 26.9 Using your right thumb, apply pressure to the first bend of the index finger of your left hand: use a rotating movement.

2 LEFT HAND – PLANTAR

The ear

Figure 26.10 Using your right thumb, apply pressure to the first bend of the third finger of your left hand: use a rotating movement.

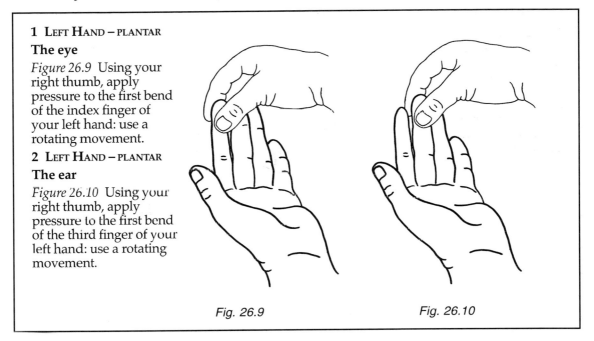

Fig. 26.9   Fig. 26.10

7 The neck and thyroid gland – (a) right hand

1 RIGHT HAND – PLANTAR
Figure 26.11
2 RIGHT HAND – DORSAL
Figure 26.12
Using the thumb of your left hand, work the reflex points found at the base of the thumb and first two fingers of your right hand. The thyroid reflex point is at the base of the thumb, but it is essential to work on the bases of the next two fingers as this helps the nerve and blood supply to the neck and you will also be able to relieve neck tension.

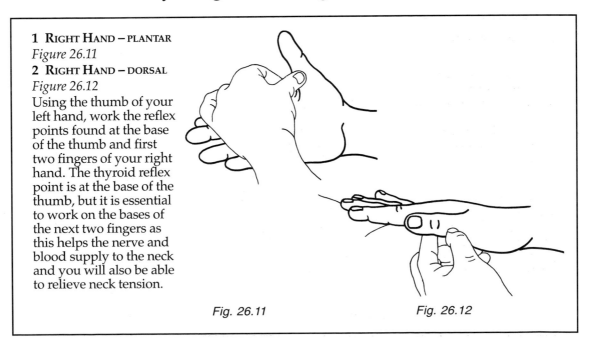

Fig. 26.11   Fig. 26.12

8 The neck and thyroid gland – (b) left hand

1 LEFT HAND – PLANTAR
Figure 26.13
2 LEFT HAND – DORSAL
Figure 26.14
Using the thumb of your right hand, work the reflex points found at the base of the thumb and first two fingers of your left hand. The thyroid reflex point is at the base of the thumb, but it is essential to work on the bases of the next two fingers as this helps the nerve and blood supply to the neck and you will also be able to relieve neck tension.

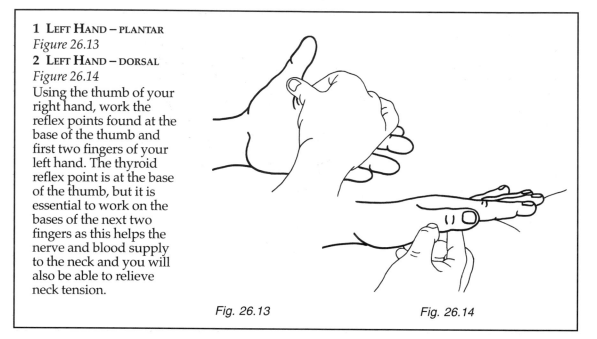

Fig. 26.13   Fig. 26.14

9 The coccyx – (a) right hand

1 RIGHT HAND – PLANTAR

Figure 26.15 To work this reflex area, apply pressure from the four fingers of your left hand to the area just in front of the thumb on the medial side of your right hand.

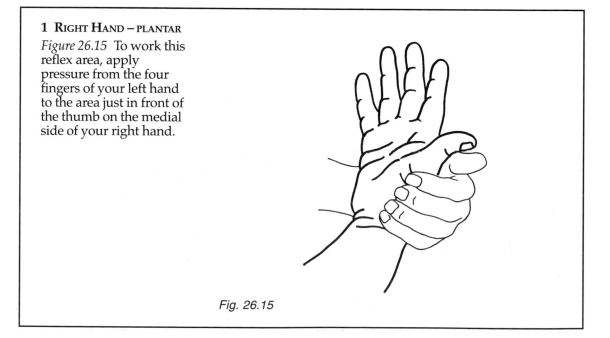

Fig. 26.15

10 The coccyx – *(b) left hand*

1 LEFT HAND – PLANTAR

Figure 26.16 To work this reflex area, apply pressure from the four fingers of your right hand to the area just in front of the thumb on the medial side of your left hand.

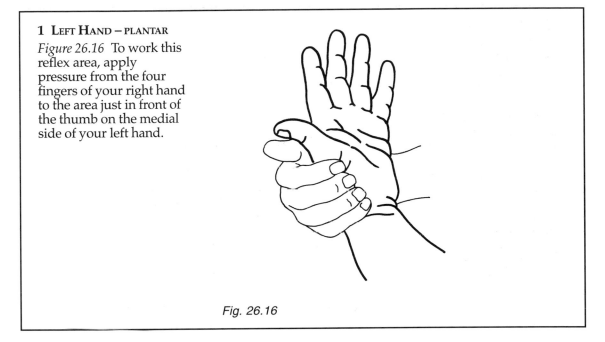

Fig. 26.16

11 The hip and pelvis – *(a) right hand*

1 RIGHT HAND – DORSAL

Figure 26.17 To work this reflex area, apply pressure from the four fingers of your left hand around the lateral side of your right hand.

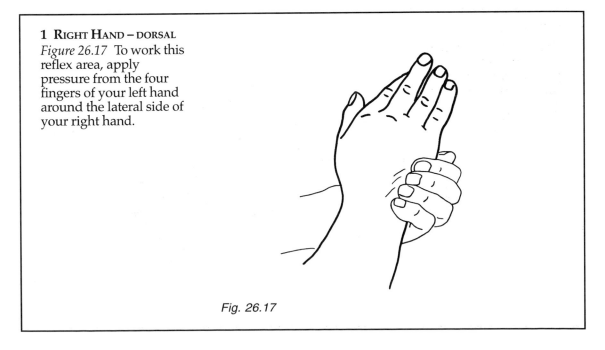

Fig. 26.17

12 The hip and pelvis – *(b) left hand*

1 LEFT HAND – DORSAL
Figure 26.18 To work this reflex area, apply pressure from the four fingers of your right hand around the lateral side of your left hand.

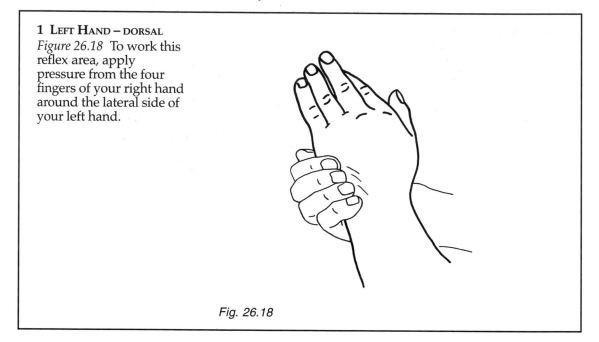

Fig. 26.18

13 The spine – *(a) right hand*

1 RIGHT HAND – PLANTAR
Figure 26.19 To contact the reflex points for the spine on your right hand, work along the line indicated with your left thumb.

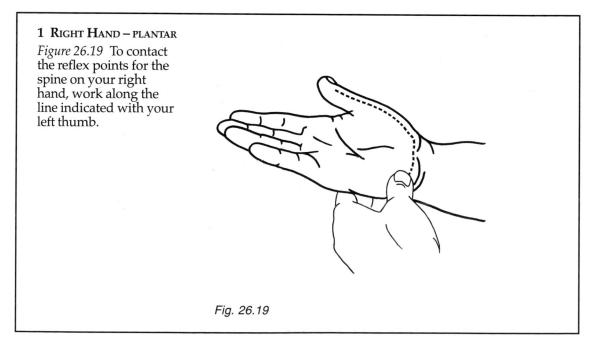

Fig. 26.19

14 The spine – *(b) left hand*

1 LEFT HAND – PLANTAR

Figure 26.20 To contact the reflex points for the spine on your left hand, work along the line indicated with your right thumb.

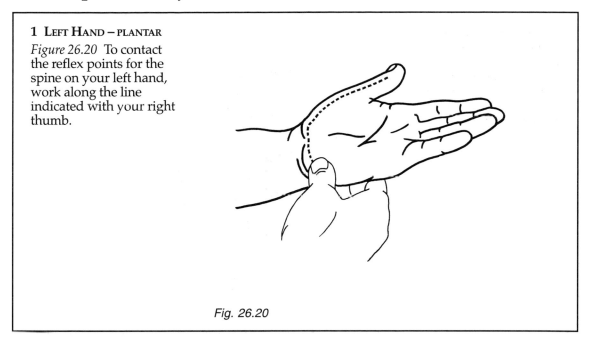

Fig. 26.20

15 The brain – *(a) right hand*

1 RIGHT HAND

Figure 26.21 To work the right side of the brain, apply pressure with the left thumb directly to the top of your right thumb.

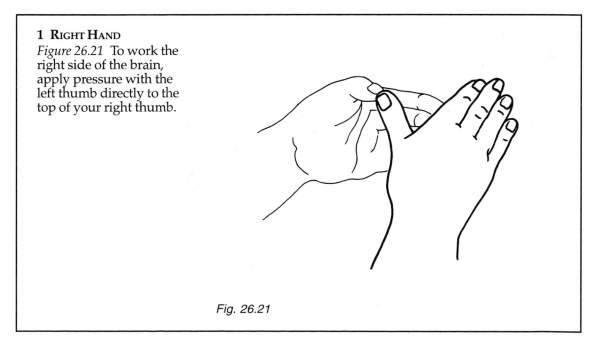

Fig. 26.21

16 The brain – *(b) left hand*

1 Left Hand

Figure 26.22 To work the left side of the brain, apply pressure with the right thumb directly to the top of your left thumb.

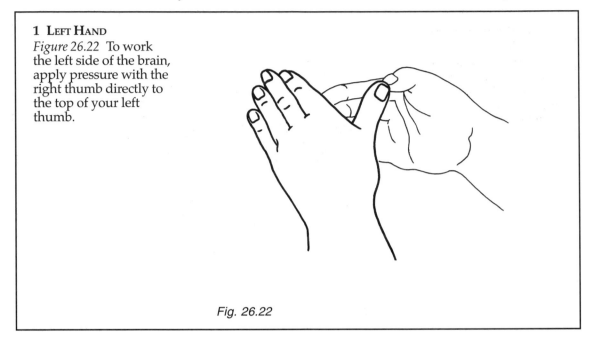

Fig. 26.22

17 The shoulder – *(a) right hand*

1 Right Hand – plantar

Figure 26.23 To work the right shoulder, apply pressure to the area indicated on your right hand using your left thumb. Repeat on your left hand to contact the reflex points for your left shoulder.

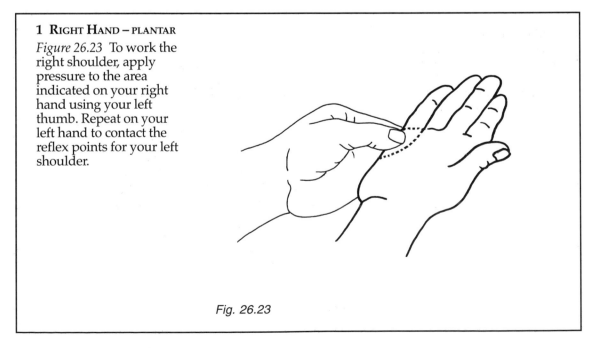

Fig. 26.23

18 The shoulder – *(b) left hand*

1 LEFT HAND – PLANTAR

Figure 26.24 To work the left shoulder, apply pressure to the area indicated on your left hand using your right thumb.

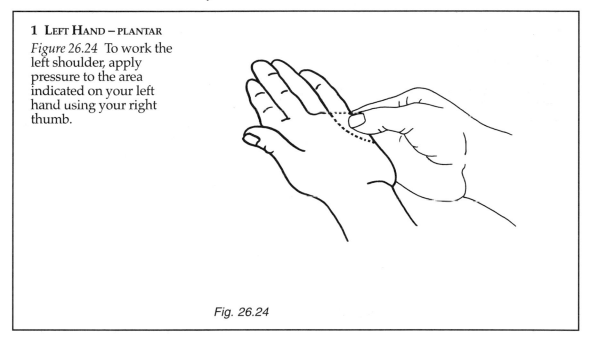

Fig. 26.24

19 The knee and elbow – *(a) right hand*

1 RIGHT HAND – DORSAL

Figure 26.25 On the right hand work out the small triangular area using the fingers of your left hand.

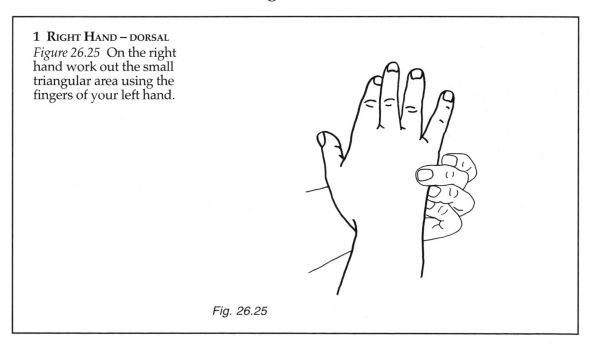

Fig. 26.25

20 The knee and elbow – *(b) left hand*

1 LEFT HAND – DORSAL
Figure 26.26 On the left hand work out the small triangular area using the fingers of your right hand.

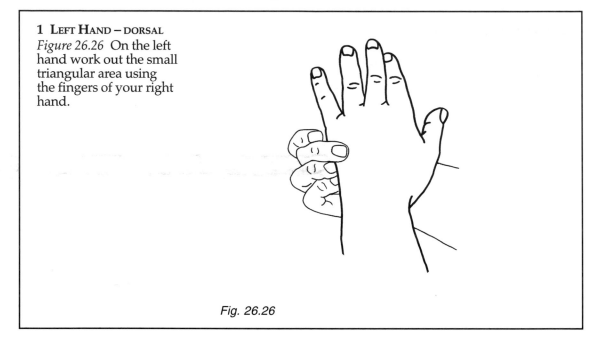

Fig. 26.26

21 The stomach, pancreas and spleen – *left hand only*

1 LEFT HAND – PLANTAR
Figure 26.27 The reflex points for these parts of the body are found only on the left hand. Use your right thumb to work over the areas indicated on your left palm.

Note The liver and gall bladder

In the same area of the right hand you will contact the reflex point for the liver and gall bladder.

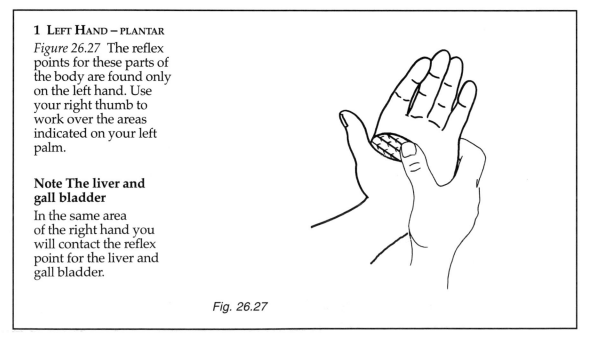

Fig. 26.27

22 The ascending, transverse and descending colon – *(a) right hand*

1 RIGHT HAND – PLANTAR

Figure 26.28 Using your left thumb, work across the palm of your right hand in the areas indicated.

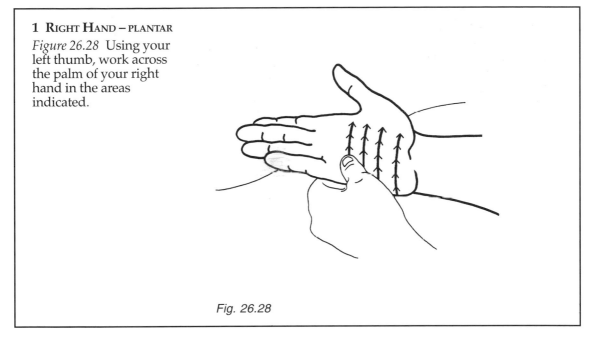

Fig. 26.28

23 The ascending, transverse and descending colon – *(b) left hand*

1 LEFT HAND – PLANTAR

Figure 26.29 Using your right thumb, work across the palm of your left hand in the areas indicated.

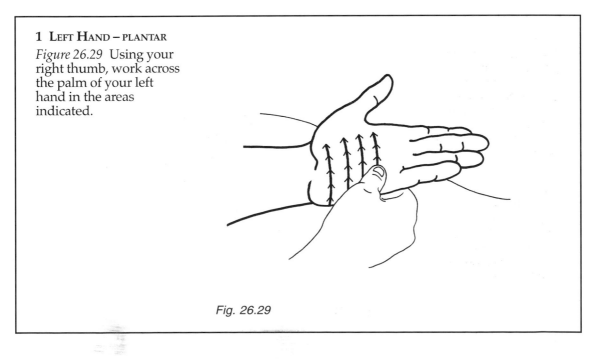

Fig. 26.29

24 The bladder – *(a) right hand*

1 RIGHT HAND – PLANTAR

Figure 26.30 Using your left thumb, apply pressure to the fleshy pad just below the thumb of your right hand.

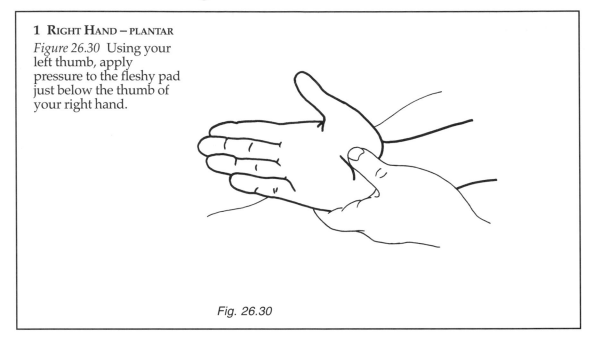

Fig. 26.30

25 The bladder – *(b) left hand*

1 LEFT HAND – PLANTAR

Figure 26.31 Using your right thumb, apply pressure to the fleshy pad just below the thumb of your left hand.

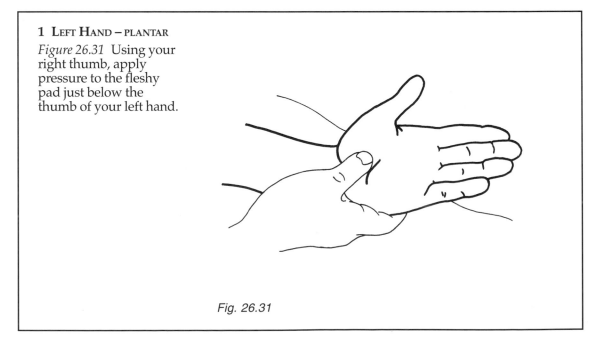

Fig. 26.31

26 The ureter tube – *(a) right hand*

1 RIGHT HAND – PLANTAR

Figure 26.32 Working the right hand with your left thumb, continue from the bladder area towards the base of your index finger.

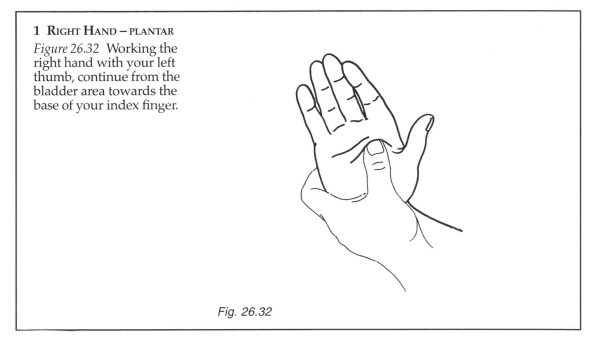

Fig. 26.32

27 The ureter tube – *(b) left hand*

1 LEFT HAND – PLANTAR

Figure 26.33 Working the left hand with your right thumb, continue from the bladder area towards the base of your index finger.

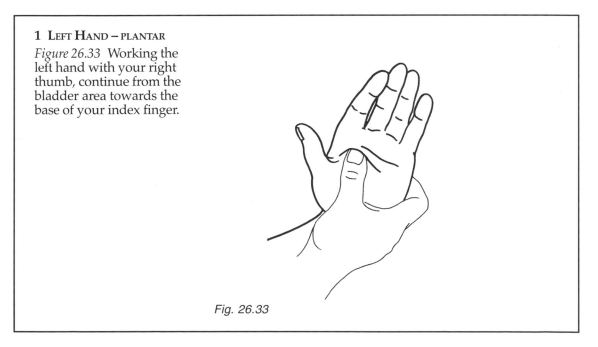

Fig. 26.33

28 The kidney – *(a) right hand*

1 RIGHT HAND – PLANTAR
Figure 26.34 Working on the right hand you will find the reflex point to the kidney just above the area to the ureter tube. Work over this point with your left thumb.

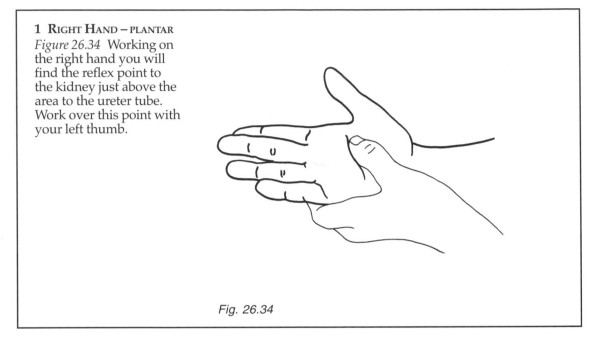

Fig. 26.34

29 The kidney – *(b) left hand*

1 LEFT HAND – PLANTAR
Figure 26.35 Working on the left hand you will find the reflex point to the kidney just above the area to the ureter tube. Work over this point with your right thumb.

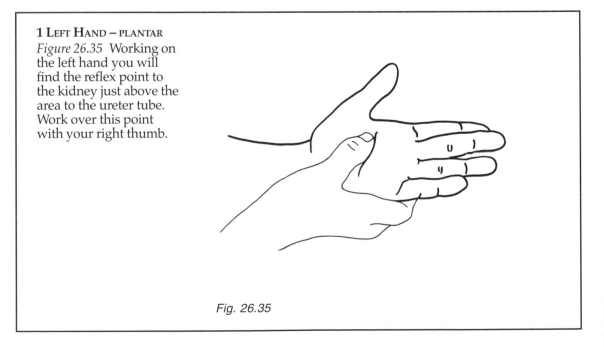

Fig. 26.35

HAND CHART

HAND CHART

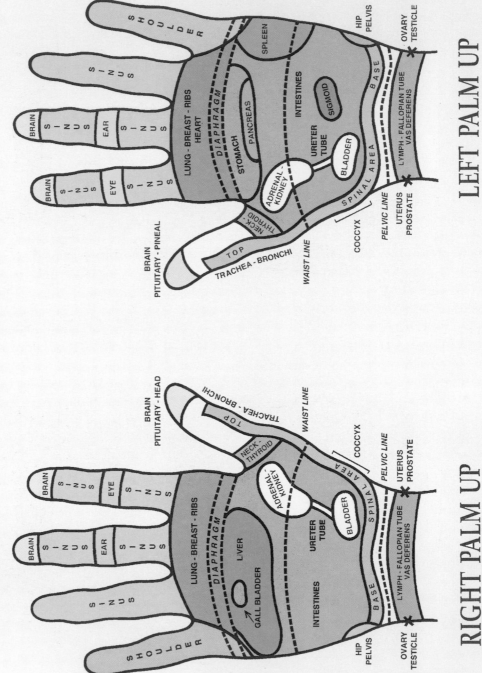

RIGHT PALM UP

LEFT PALM UP

Left hand labels:

BRAIN
PITUITARY - PINEAL

BRAIN

SINUS

SINUS

EAR

SINUS

EYE

SINUS

SINUS

SHOULDER

SPLEEN

HIP
PELVIS

OVARY
TESTICLE

LUNG - BREAST - RIBS
HEART

DIAPHRAGM

STOMACH

PANCREAS

INTESTINES

SIGMOID

BASE

ADRENAL -
KIDNEY

URETER
TUBE

BLADDER

SPINAL AREA

NECK -
THYROID

TOP

TRACHEA - BRONCHI

WAIST LINE

COCCYX

PELVIC LINE

UTERUS
PROSTATE

SPINAL AREA

LYMPH - FALLOPIAN TUBE
VAS DEFERENS

Right hand labels:

BRAIN
PITUITARY - HEAD

BRAIN

SINUS

EYE

SINUS

BRAIN

SINUS

EAR

SINUS

SINUS

SHOULDER

TOP

TRACHEA - BRONCHI

NECK -
THYROID

WAIST LINE

LUNG - BREAST - RIBS

DIAPHRAGM

LIVER

GALL BLADDER

ADRENAL -
KIDNEY

URETER
TUBE

BLADDER

INTESTINES

SPINAL AREA

COCCYX

PELVIC LINE

UTERUS
PROSTATE

BASE

HIP
PELVIS

OVARY
TESTICLE

LYMPH - FALLOPIAN TUBE
VAS DEFERENS

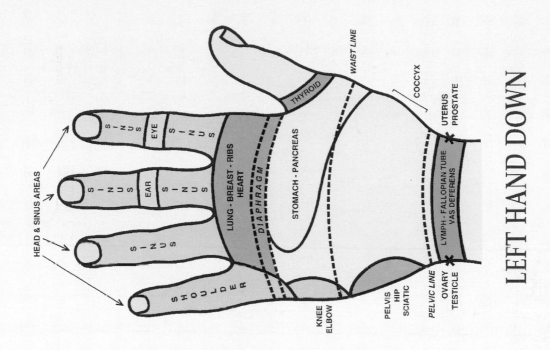

LEFT HAND DOWN

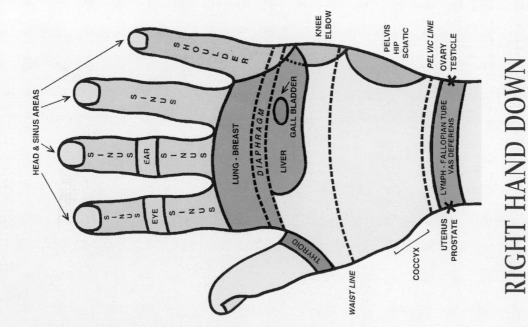

RIGHT HAND DOWN

30 The uterus/prostate – *(a) right hand*

1 RIGHT HAND – PLANTAR

Figure 26.36 Using the third finger of your left hand make contact with and work out the reflex points on the area of your wrist below the thumb.

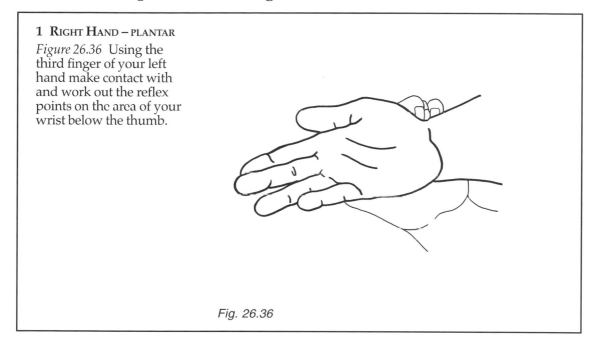

Fig. 26.36

31 The uterus/prostate – *(b) left hand*

1 LEFT HAND – PLANTAR

Figure 26.37 Using the third finger of your right hand make contact with and work out the reflex points on the area of your wrist below the thumb.

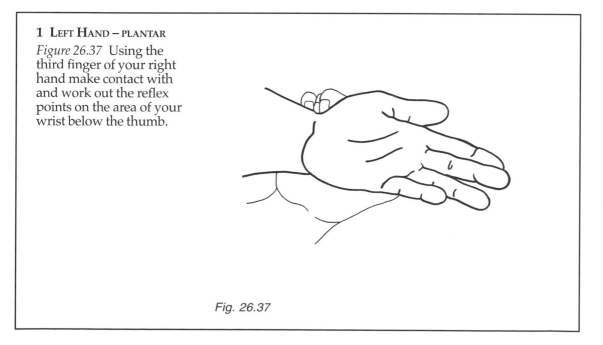

Fig. 26.37

32 The ovaries/testes – *(a) right hand*

1 RIGHT HAND – DORSAL

Figure 26.38 Use the third finger of your left hand to contact and work the reflex point just in front of your right wrist bone.

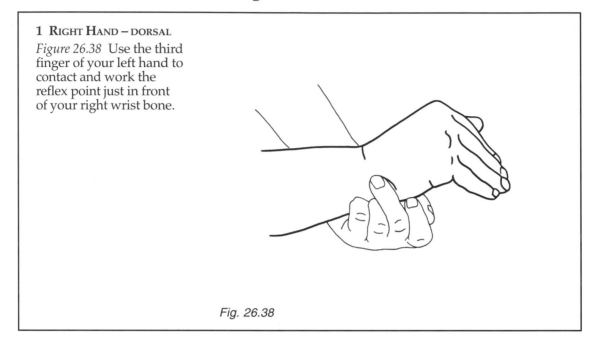

Fig. 26.38

33 The ovaries/testes – *(b) left hand*

1 LEFT HAND – DORSAL

Figure 26.39 Use the third finger of your right hand to contact and work the reflex point just in front of your left wrist bone.

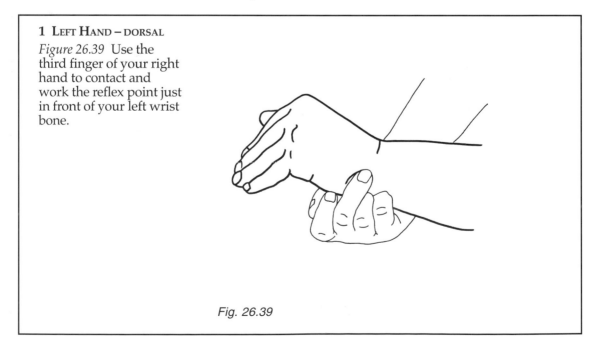

Fig. 26.39

34 Fallopian tubes/Vas deferens – *(a) right hand*

1 RIGHT HAND – PLANTAR

Figure 26.40 Applying pressure from all four fingers of your left hand, work out the area across the top of the wrist.

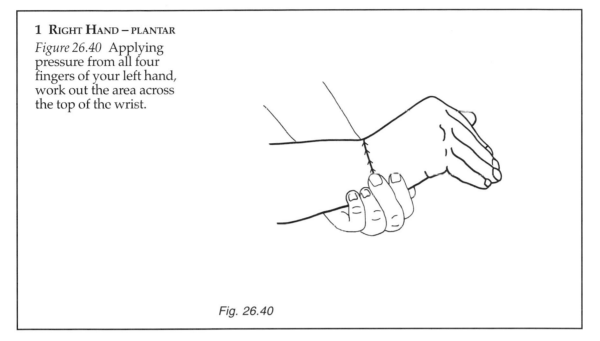

Fig. 26.40

35 Fallopian tubes/Vas deferens – *(b) left hand*

1 LEFT HAND – PLANTAR

Figure 26.41 Applying pressure from all four fingers of your right hand, work out the area across the top of the wrist.

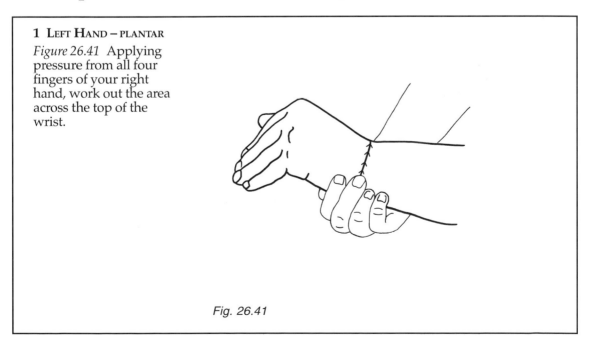

Fig. 26.41

CHAPTER 27 Hand relaxation exercises

Hand relaxation exercises are special techniques that are used at the beginning of a treatment session, during a treatment and at the end of the session.

The principle is very similar to giving a foot reflexology treatment in as much as the exercises relax the hand and create a contact between patient and practitioner.

If you sit facing your patient with their arm and hand resting on a table which will be between you, and place the arm on a large pillow so that good support is given, this will be the best position to start your treatment.

1 Side-to-side relaxation

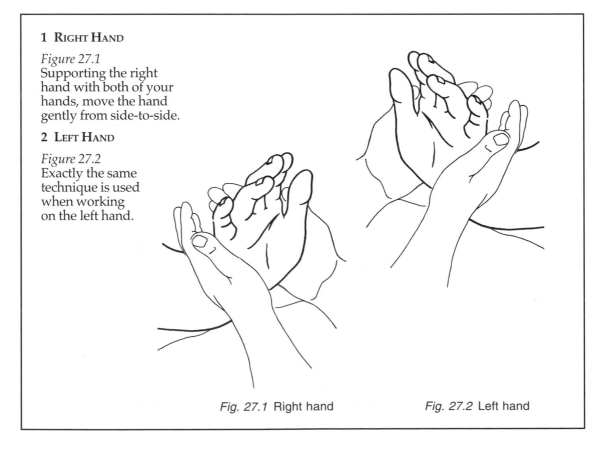

1 RIGHT HAND

Figure 27.1
Supporting the right hand with both of your hands, move the hand gently from side-to-side.

2 LEFT HAND

Figure 27.2
Exactly the same technique is used when working on the left hand.

Fig. 27.1 Right hand   *Fig. 27.2* Left hand

2 Metacarpal kneading

1 RIGHT HAND

Figures 27.3 and 27.4
Supporting the right hand with your left hand, make a fist with your right hand and use it to knead the receiver's palm.

2 LEFT HAND

Figures 27.5 and 27.6
Repeat this exercise for the left hand, using your right hand as a support and making a fist with your left hand.

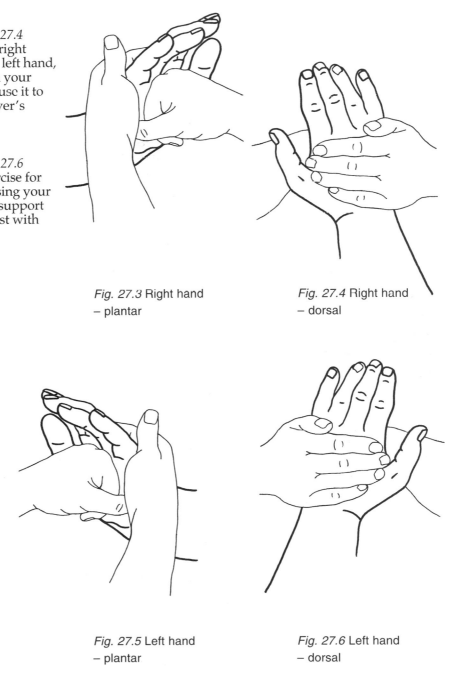

Fig. 27.3 Right hand – plantar

Fig. 27.4 Right hand – dorsal

Fig. 27.5 Left hand – plantar

Fig. 27.6 Left hand – dorsal

3 Diaphragm relaxation

1 RIGHT HAND

This exercise helps to relax the large diaphragm muscle which is found at the base of the lung.

Figure 27.7 Place your thumb on the diaphragm line and gently bend the fingers over on to your thumb. Move your right thumb along this line from the medial to the lateral edge.

2 LEFT HAND

Figure 27.8 Repeat this exercise for the left hand.

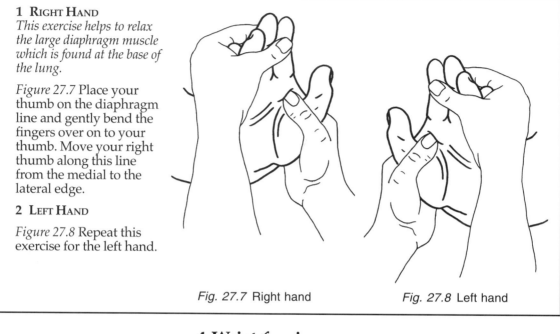

Fig. 27.7 Right hand   Fig. 27.8 Left hand

4 Wrist freeing

1 RIGHT HAND

Figure 27.9 Supporting the right hand in front of the wrist, with the heels of both your hands, rock the hand from side-to-side.

2 LEFT HAND

Figure 27.10 Repeat this exercise for the left hand.

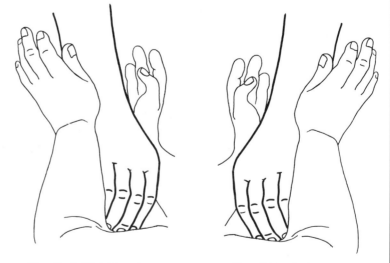

Fig. 27.9 Right hand   Fig. 27.10 Left hand

5 Undergrip

1 RIGHT HAND

Figure 27.11 Supporting with the left hand, turn the hand inwards in a rotating direction.

2 LEFT HAND

Figure 27.12 Repeat this exercise for the left hand.

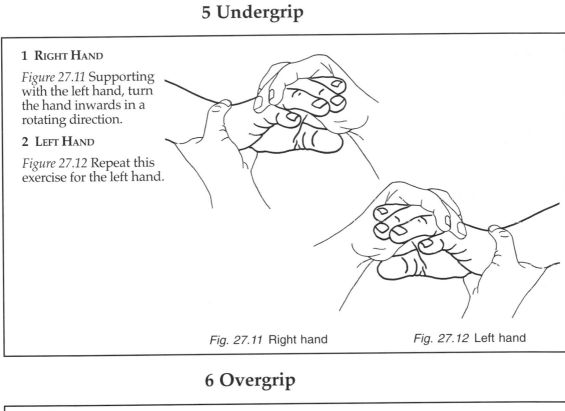

Fig. 27.11 Right hand   Fig. 27.12 Left hand

6 Overgrip

1 RIGHT HAND

Figure 27.13 Support the right hand by placing your left hand over the top of the wrist and use your right hand to turn the hand inward.

2 LEFT HAND

Figure 27.14 Repeat this exercise for the left hand.

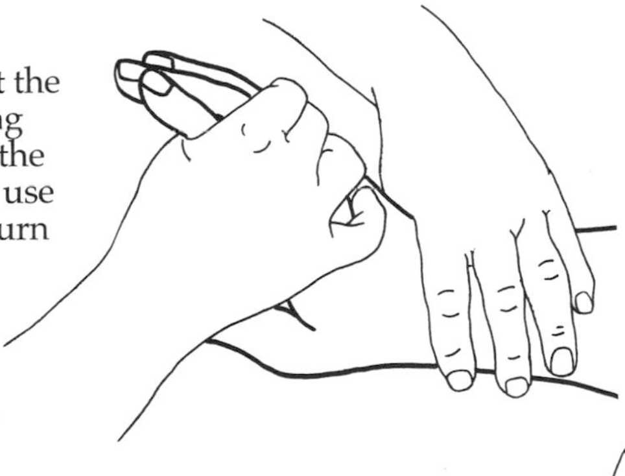

Fig. 27.13 Right hand 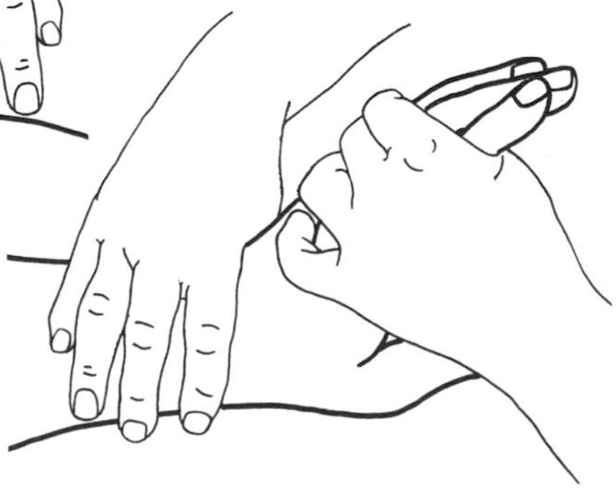   Fig. 27.14 Left hand

7 Hand moulding

1 RIGHT HAND

Figure 27.15 Cradle the right hand in the palms of your hands and from the lateral side of the hand, rotate.

2 LEFT HAND

Figure 27.16 Repeat this exercise for the left hand.

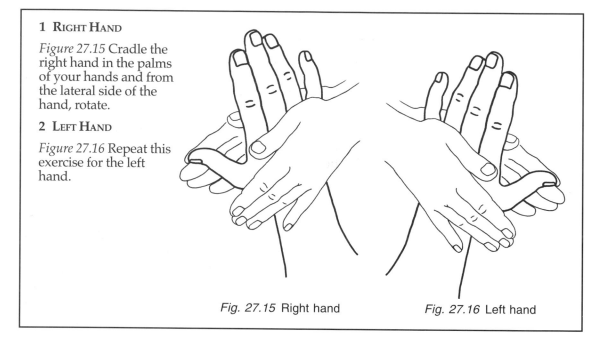

Fig. 27.15 Right hand *Fig. 27.16* Left hand

8 Rib cage relaxation

1 RIGHT HAND

Figure 27.17 Working on the right hand, press in with the thumbs of both of your hands and creep around the dorsal side of the hand with the four free fingers of each hand.

2 LEFT HAND

Figure 27.18 Repeat this exercise for the left hand.

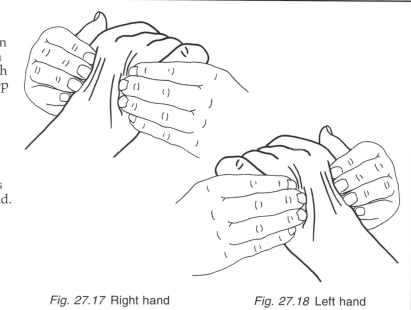

Fig. 27.17 Right hand *Fig. 27.18* Left hand

CHAPTER **28** # Don't blame it on the weather

The poor old British weather gets the blame for most of our aches and pains, sniffles and sneezes. We proclaim that, if we sit in a draught or go out in the wind or get exposed to low temperatures, we are going to catch colds or 'flu.

There again we still grumble when it is hot, because we then say that germs and viruses absolutely thrive in the heat causing 'summer colds', gastro-intestinal infections and the like.

The real causes of illness

Generally speaking the weather is not the cause of illness. The cause of disease is when the body fails to eliminate all of its toxic wastes from the liver, the kidneys, the lungs, the intestines and the skin. In such circumstances we have an overloaded system; viruses and bacteria thrive in this destructive element. It was Louis Pasteur who proclaimed, 'Don't worry about the viruses, worry about the soil in which they grow'. So if the soil is right disease flourishes.

It is very common to hear of some epidemic early in the New Year and then it is always blamed on the grey dark dismal days of January, cold temperatures, high winds and the damp environment. Although looking out on to this type of grey day is not very stimulating to the mind and certainly does not make us feel at our best, it is still not the main cause of illness.

More than likely the main cause of an infectious spread of anything is simply because after Christmas and into the New Year we have done an enormous amount of indulging in very high calorie fat and carbohydrate based foods and our alcohol intake has probably been higher than at any time of the year. Consequently our bodies are totally clogged and congested and are having a struggle to eliminate all their waste efficiently. We then find that the virus or bacteria which attacks us and gives us a bout of 'flu, gastric 'flu or a heavy cold is simply the result of over-

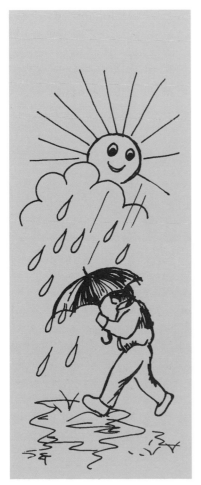

indulgence through the Christmas period.

The air around us and the rain are good for the body; they are good for the skin, and fresh air never did anything but revitalise and improve our circulatory and respiratory function. Why then do we, the British, always look for the cause of illness in an external environment?

Disease is created from within, never from without. Apart from the exceptional circumstances when people in under-developed countries are living on inadequate supplies of food and in areas where there is open sewerage so that dysentery and cholera are rife, our health should be unaffected by weather conditions.

You may find that when you have some epidemic in your office, it is not every single member of staff who goes down with the illness. Although the viruses must be multiplying in their billions in the warm surroundings of an office where numbers of people are working together in the same place, it does not necessarily follow that the illness will affect everyone.

There could be one member of staff who, whatever happens, does not go down with Asian 'flu or something similar, and that is because that person's body is in a far less congested state than others.

Disease also manifests when we are in a low mental state; when our interest in life has declined; when we feel we have no real function, purpose, or direction. Maybe we are suffering from a very painful recent loss of a member of our family. Our immune system will be greatly affected by negative emotional feelings of this kind, and it is normal that when a person is under stress they will find that their health deteriorates, and that they fall prey to almost any illness around.

I am sure you have heard it said, 'I seem to catch everything that is going around'. All that antibiotics and drugs do is simply to suppress the symptoms. Remember, you still have the underlying cause, the congested body, so until you resolve this you are very likely to have a recurrence within a week or two.

Sometimes a respiratory infection is severe and seriously affects breathing and we do have to resort to taking antibiotics, but it is quite common to find that a couple of weeks later you have an episode of diarrhoea and sickness. This is the body's way of trying to get rid of the congestion which is still there.

A purpose to life

I remember a very moving story told to me at a meeting I attended recently, quoted from a book *'Man's Search for a Meaning'* by Victor Frankel.

Victor was one of the prisoners in the death camps in Germany during the last war. Within a few months of being taken to the camp he saw the atrocities that occurred within, and despite his weak, painfully thin body, he decided that he was going to try to survive because he wanted to be able to write about the experiences he saw, so that never again could these terrible things happen to man. So you see, Victor had a real purpose for living.

Confined to his cell Victor wrote about the experiences he witnessed. Of course, had any of the notes which he wrote been discovered, he would have been instantly put to death, but somehow he managed to hide his papers and keep this very vital information secret.

One day he was taken with a hundred other prisoners into the dreaded gas chambers and he felt sure that this was the end. To his and the other prisoners' amazement, when the jets were switched on above them they found that it was not gas, it was ice cold water that came out of them. These prisoners, naked men, were standing under these ice cold jets in sub-zero temperatures for hours. Remember that they were all in a terrible state of emaciation and were just mere skin and bone; some had a lot of sores and scarring to the body from mutilation and torture, but, as Frankel said in his book, the joy of experiencing this ice cold water rather than choking gas was more than he would ever have expected, because here there was hope. He was not going to die on this particular day; he had a purpose to survive to tell the tale, and was still alive.

During the hours of exposure icicles formed and hung on the naked bodies of all the prisoners. Icicles attached themselves to their noses, fingers and any extremities that they could get a hold on and somehow they still survived. Then the water was turned off. Many of the prisoners had frozen together. Nevertheless they were returned to their cells and not one single person from those hundred prisoners contracted pneumonia, a cold, or 'flu or anything else.

The reason was that they were so determined to survive and they were so exhilarated by receiving cold water rather than toxic gases into their bodies, that their life force was stimulated at their chance, at the very smallest chance of survival.

Over the next weeks most of the prisoners who went through that torturous episode were gassed. However, Victor was one who did survive and lived to write the book from which I am quoting this story and, despite the most terrible ill-health, the torture, the damage to his body and the emaciation, he did survive and he survived because he had real purpose and direction – a search for meaning.

How then can it possibly be that we, who are living in such a comfortable environment as most of us do today, with heating, lighting, plenty of food, fresh air (although I must confess that it has become more polluted of latter years), and with some sort of income, even if sparse, can then blame all our aches and pains on to the weather?

If you read this chapter again you will perhaps better understand how it is the mind that has the greatest influence on whether or not you survive ordeals that may come your way.

The importance of family

People who are loved, wanted and supported and are within a close partnership have far more chance of survival from any traumatic episode in their life than solitary individuals who perhaps have lost all their main family and are living in a lone state.

Every developmental stage of life poses some degree

of physical and psychological challenge. The most dependant stage of life is infancy, but to some extent we all depend on each other throughout our life. We depend on those responsible for our electricity supply to do their job, otherwise we would be sorely affected by the absence of this power. We depend on those working to control the flow of water through our reservoirs in order that we have a constant supply of water in our homes: we would all be seriously affected if our water supply ceased.

In our adult life dependency needs are usually fulfilled by a close relationship but should the relationship break down, insecurities may emerge which encourage us to eat and drink too much, take up things like smoking and gambling and this neglect of our health results in all the stress related illnesses: peptic ulcers, indigestion, irritable bowel syndrome and attacks of disabling migraine. These are the common symptoms experienced by adults when going through a divorce or bereavement, which result in feelings of rage, depression, anger, confusion and apprehension, with demands for instant solutions to the problems which resurface at this time.

Pregnancy

Pregnancy is a time of life which needs major physical and psychological adjustments, particularly to the mother who not only is responsible for providing the nurturing and nourishment to the unborn child for 40 weeks, but will provide the nest into which her baby will arrive and flourish. These changes exert a great deal of pressure on the mother who may have other children to care for.

Fathers go through psychological changes too and may develop symptoms associated with pregnancy: nausea, resembling morning sickness, and mood swings.

The hormonal changes during pregnancy are enormous, and these often account for mood swings from feelings of depression and anxiety, to elation. There may exist feelings of doubts as to whether the mother will be able to cope with the physical and emotional trauma of birth; whether giving birth will proceed normally; whether unexpected complications will arise. These anxieties are not at all unusual. Happily most women have a normal pregnancy which leads to the delivery of a healthy baby.

The menopause

The menopause affects women from about 40 onwards and is a period of both physical and emotional adjustment. The classic symptoms of apprehension, sweating and palpitations are some of the more common discomforts. Perhaps the main area to consider is the role of the glands during the menopausal years. Until the menopause the ovaries are the primary site of oestrogen production. After this time, when the supply of egg bearing follicles have become depleted, the ovaries become unable to release oestrogen and, although signals continue to be stimulated from the pituitary and hypothalamus which are the master glands of the endocrine system often referred to as 'the master of the orchestra', the release of oestrogen is not forthcoming which must create some biological confusion.

However, the ovaries are not the only glands which produce sex hormones. The adrenal glands, sitting on top of both kidneys like a small cap, manufacture oestrogens and androgens (male hormones), the latter being responsible for the sex drive in women as well as men. It depends on the health of our adrenal glands as to whether they will be able to take over the production of hormones efficiently. Coffee drinking in excess and alcohol, plus a stressful life, cause adrenal exhaustion. Not only do our adrenal glands produce sex hormones, they are responsible for many other functions and the following list shows the demand that is made on these two tiny glands.

1 The adrenal glands regulate blood sugar levels, along with the pancreas.

2 They help dissipate any inflammatory or allergic reaction in the body.

3 They are also responsible for the regulation of salt and potassium levels.

Alcohol and smoking are the two main substances that should be avoided if the woman is going through a difficult time with the menopause. One of the key benefits in setting up an appropriate diet for the menopausal years is to consume foods with the highest level of nutrients and the lowest level of what are known as 'wasted calories' which have a poor nutritional value: white sugar and white flour products in particular, and a diet that has a high animal fat content.

The B vitamins, especially vitamin B6, vitamin C and vitamins E and D are important. Make sure you are taking sufficient minerals: zinc, magnesium and calcium in particular. Whole grains, especially brown rice, brown bread, oats, barley and corn, are all to be recommended, and at least five pieces of fruit and three or more vegetables every day.

During our menstruating years we are less likely to suffer from coronary heart disease, or osteoporosis, as the constant supply of oestrogen and progesterone act as a preventative. Once our ovaries reduce the supply of oestrogen, we then become more susceptible to the diseases of circulation and our bones become more brittle.

Mood swings are very common at this time as for some, the cessation of the periods marks the beginning of 'old age'. For many, the freedom from the monthly discomfort plus a time of life when most children have fled the nest and become independent, marks a new beginning; a time to take things at a slower pace and maybe take up new interests. So many women have found that their postmenopausal years have been the best years of their life.

The elderly

Problems occur in the elderly because they become physically and emotionally stiff and rigid.

The physical disabilities make the everyday routines of life wearing and frustrating: stiff wrists find it hard to unscrew bottles and jars and stiff, painful hips make bending and lifting almost impossible. Consequently, the efforts in dealing with simple household tasks bring to the surface emotions such as anger, depression and despair.

Like the child the elderly person is vulnerable to heat, cold and fluctuations in temperature. Many of the common circulatory disorders which occur at this time are either associated with a diminished body surface or impaired temperature regulatory mechanism.

The need to feel safe and secure in their own home is understandable – that familiar chair, or the comfort of their own bed, and a kitchen where the pots and pans are easily accessible give the elderly a special sense of security – so a trip to relatives or friends often causes a sense of panic.

The warden-assisted accommodation for the elderly is often the solution when managing every day domesticities becomes impossible. Any emergencies can be dealt with and the company and social contact with other elderly people help dispel the feelings of loneliness.

Cancer and coronary heart disease

The main purpose of this book is to give theoretical instruction of reflexology but since cancer and coronary heart disease are the two diseases which cause highest mortality in the developed world, I have chosen to write about these two illnesses in depth: they can both be helped considerably with attention to diet, lifestyle, vitamin and mineral support and, of course, reflexology.

CHAPTER **29** Understanding cancer

The very word fills most of us with dread. We feel as if a death sentence had just been imposed. At the commencement of this century cancer was responsible for taking the life of one person in 30. Today, it claims the life of one in five. One in three of us in the West will have cancer at some time in our lives and it is unfortunately the way that most of us will die.

Very little is known about cancer. We have made little progress in the treatment of it and certainly are no further forward in understanding the cause.

Cancer is basically a disease of affluence, hence the main reason for the increase in the last 30 years. All the billions of dollars thrown at research has not influenced the survival rate one little bit. How could it, if today one person in every five is dying from it?

Let us look at our lifestyles. Most of us live in an environment that the human body was not expected to cope with.

Our environment
Pollution
We are bombarded with pollution from every angle from the increased traffic on our roads, and there is no possibility that this will decrease in the future. Air traffic increases by the year adding even more pollution to our atmosphere. Chemical leakages from factories cause disasters to our water and again, pollute the air which we breathe. We spray our fields with chemicals that were not meant to be used on this planet, let alone be ingested into our bodies through the food that we eat. We spray our fruit trees in order that the housewife sees perfect fruit on the supermarket shelf: all these chemicals create changes in our bodies.

We are surrounded by machinery in our homes. Have you ever stopped to think that your washing machine, heated dryer, microwave, dishwasher, hair dryer, all these devices, give off a certain amount of electromagnetic energy. We have all read of the claims that have been made by those who have been unfortunate enough to live near power lines which have caused children to contract leukaemia. It is a fact that living near power lines can raise the chance of your child getting this disease by three or four times.

Flouridated water

An American Government study has confirmed that fluoride added to water caused cancer in laboratory animals: cancers of the liver, bone and mouth were found.

Drugs

Cholesterol-controlling drugs

There has been a link with cancer and drugs used to reduce cholesterol levels. Every attempt should be made to reduce cholesterol levels the natural way: reduce animal fats like the plague; eat no more than four ounces of red meat with a meal and then no more than two red meat meals per week. Reduce alcohol consumption to the absolute minimum and take up some form of regular exercise to encourage the body to burn up the fat content of the liver.

Fertility drugs

There are links with these drugs and ovarian and breast cancer. Many cases of infertility can be rectified by taking specific minerals and vitamins and following a good diet, and any nutritional expert will guide you in this direction, if this is what you wish. It is always best to try natural, simple methods first and leave drug therapies as an absolute last resort.

Cervical cancer

Certain nutritional deficiencies can increase the risk of developing cervical cancer: women deficient in folic acid are more likely to have cervical abnormalities. Other risk factors are: smoking, having a variety of sexual partners particularly in the teenage years when the cervix is immature, and an excessive consumption of alcohol.

A 1988 study showed that nearly half of smears with mild abnormalities reverted to normal within two years. None of the patients developed invasive cancer during long-term follow-up. (BMJ 1988.297; 18-21).

Even a simple inflammation of the cervix can show up as an abnormal smear!

Smoking

There is absolutely no doubt at all that smoking causes cancer. 89 per cent of lung cancers would disappear if we could no longer get hold of cigarettes. Whether or not you smoke cigarettes, a pipe, cigars, or 'roll your own', the tar and the chemicals in the tobacco cause the cancer and the nicotine creates the addiction.

Smoking encourages the growth of cancer in all parts of your body: your mouth, your throat, stomach, intestines, prostate, pancreas, uterus, ovaries – every part of the human body – because no part of the body is separated from the other. The human body is an entity and every organ or function depends on all being in tune so that this miraculous human machine can remain healthy and active.

Hormone replacement therapy (HRT)

There is no doubt that this drug can increase your breast cancer risk by 60 per cent in those taking the drug for more than five years.

High fat diets

A link has been shown with those taking a high fat diet and, in particular, colon cancer. It is also a contributing factor in most cancers.

Since the introduction of vast changes in the eating habits of the nation in the last 20 years, which encourages the consumption of chips with almost everything, beefburgers, hamburgers, take-away meals and pizzas, to name just a few items of food on the menu of most families, cancer has increased manifoldly, and so has our weight.

During the war years when we all lived on very sparse rations, particularly where proteins and fats were concerned, we were much thinner, and certainly statistics show that we were never in fact so healthy. Added to the sparsity of our diets maybe the support and friendship we received from our neighbours were two contributing factors in the statistics of the state of our health, and people were more concerned with the survival of their loved ones who were away fighting for our Country rather than worrying about material possessions, which probably were the last thing on anybody's mind at the time. Added to this we all walked more, as cars were an absolute luxury, and so took far more exercise.

X-rays

The frequent use of X-rays increases your exposure to radiation which in turn increases your chances of developing cancer, and dental X-rays are included in this.

Vaccinations

Although they do have their place, we really are going over the top in vaccinating our children against everything.

Why do children have childhood illnesses like measles, mumps, chickenpox and German measles in their early years? They contract these illnesses because they were meant to have them. The only way the immune system learns what to do when the invasion of bacteria or a virus attacks the system, is to have 'some lessons'. These illnesses stimulate the immune system to work efficiently.

When you have a childhood illness you are usually protected for the rest of your life against ever having it again. You do not get this lifelong protection from a vaccination – they do have to be repeated throughout your life.

Could it not be, therefore, that when a cancer cell appears on the scene, the body is so supported by vaccination that it does not know how to cope with the cancer cell!? Maybe this is the reason for the large increase in tumours in young children plus the other contributory factors that we have dealt with in this chapter.

Stress

There is no doubt that stress is yet another contributing factor in the cause of cancer. Bereavement, divorce, redundancy, the enforced move to a new area away from friends and relatives, drug taking in our children, sexual abuse; all these stresses can encourage the development of cancer, why? Simply because stress depletes our immune system.

We use up huge amounts of our life-energy when we are stressed and our poor old immune system is one of the first systems to suffer.

Never before have we had so much terminal disease – so despite the introduction of billions of tons of drugs for treating cancer, we really have not made any great steps forward.

Many people have tried alternative treatments for cancer and many have been successful in having a better quality of life for the years that they did live.

What can we do to help ourselves?

There is no way that we can all jump off this planet and seek our refuge in pastures new, nor can we as individuals do much to control the pollution which ultimately is having a devastating effect on the ozone layer, but we can, with a little personal effort, do much to improve the life that we have.

• Do change your eating habits, if they mainly contain the high fat, fast foods that are advertised and encouraged today. Good eating does not have to be expensive; fruit and vegetables are cheap enough, particularly if they are bought from local markets rather than in our supermarkets where we pay almost twice the price for most of them.

• Do reserve a time in your week for some form of enjoyable exercise, whether it be an hour or two in the local gym, a swim, an aerobics class, or just a brisk walk with your dog. Make time. Your body likes to be activated.

• Do take a multi-vitamin tablet, and if you are prone to infections of the chest or nose, include garlic and vitamin C: these help the body fight off infection.

• Do drink plenty of water. We need to constantly flush out our systems with water; this helps the body eliminate toxins.

• Give up smoking. It is hard, but it can be done if you really have to want to kick the habit.

- Take your alcohol in small quantities. It is better to have a glass of wine a day than indulge in a large intake on one specific day. The liver cannot cope with large quantities of alcohol at any one time, and you may well cause some of the liver cells to die.
- Don't be tempted to take on that bigger mortgage in order to get a much larger house if you really do not need one. This will ultimately result in much larger bills. The stress of huge financial commitments can place such a burden on relationships, take the fun out of life and make you ill at ease – dis-ease – which is at the root of all illness.
- Try not to harbour grudges and make an effort to find a nice thing to say about everybody you meet. Very few of us do not have something pleasant in our personalities!
- Don't bottle up your feelings: express them openly and honestly. Unexpressed emotions create havoc in our bodies.

THE MAIN AREAS TO TREAT IN HELPING THE PATIENT WITH CANCER.

Working the digestive system

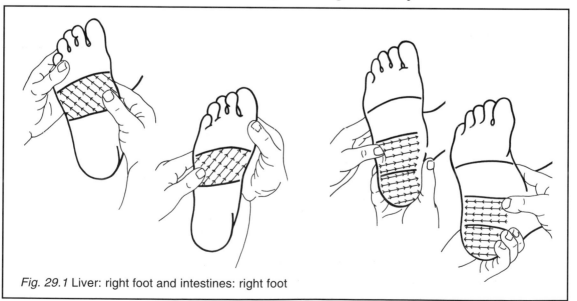

Fig. 29.1 Liver: right foot and intestines: right foot

Working the digestive system continued

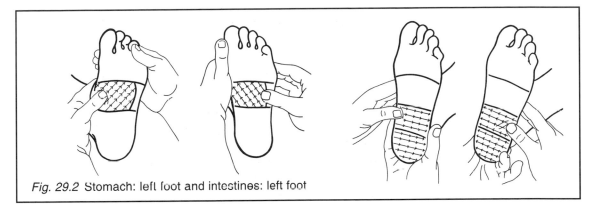

Fig. 29.2 Stomach: left foot and intestines: left foot

Working the lymphatic system – the spleen

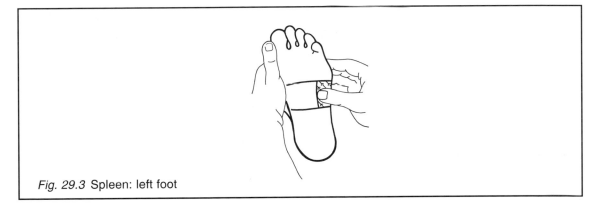

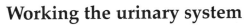

Fig. 29.3 Spleen: left foot

Working the urinary system

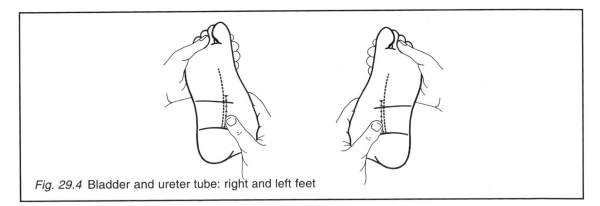

Fig. 29.4 Bladder and ureter tube: right and left feet

CHAPTER **30** Coronary heart disease

Atherosclerosis, or hardening of the arteries which eventually leads to coronary heart disease is the major cause of death, particularly amongst males; in fact it has reached almost epidemic proportions in the western world.

Heart attacks account for 20 per cent of all deaths in the US whilst degenerative and arteriosclerotic heart disease accounts for 33 per cent. Diseased arteries in the brain, which ultimately lead to a stroke, are the third most common cause of death.

Nobody was ever 'such a fit person' and then suffered a heart attack. We hear this said all the time. Atherosclerosis is a degenerative condition of the arteries which begins very, very early in life, as far back as early childhood. It is the building of atheromatous plaque in the wall of the arteries that starts the narrowing process, and is just like the plumbing system of a house; when corrosion occurs in the pipes the amount of water supply is diminished, the flow reduces as the corrosion builds leaving a smaller and smaller space for the water to flow.

Exactly the same procedure occurs within our bodies: less and less space is allowed for the blood to flow unimpeded through our arteries and veins, so the heart has to work harder and harder to pump the blood through the congested arteries.

The corrosion of our arteries is such a silent disease and that is the problem. We are often unaware that anything is wrong until it is too late and we have a sudden heart attack, unfortunately often a fatal one. The same problem arises with hypertension, you may be totally unaware that you have high blood pressure until you attend for a medical and the levels are found to be well above normal limits. Hypertension is often referred to as the 'silent killer'.

Maybe that uncomfortable feeling in your chest which you confused for indigestion, or that dizzy feeling in your head, or laboured feeling in your legs really was a signal, a cry from the body, that all was not right, and which you unfortunately ignored.

Not only does the corroded artery impede blood flow to the heart but because of a reduction in blood flow, clots are more likely to form. Think of your circulation in its healthy state as a fast flowing stream with all the twigs and stones being bounded along with the flow. Diseased arteries cause a stagnant blood flow, rather like the limited movement of the water in a stagnant pond.

If you are a smoker, the problems are immense as the sticky tar deposits in tobacco cause a sticky lining to the arterial wall, an invitation therefore for a small clot to adhere to the artery wall and cause a heart attack or stroke.

We all know that if coronary artery disease is familial in your family it increases the risks, particularly in males, of the illness occurring. However, we can either all sit down and do nothing and wait for the end to come or tackle the problem and do just everything we possibly can to avoid the disease.

Swallowing doctors' pills may help but they are not the answer. If they were the answer the death rates from heart disease would not be so high. Most sufferers are taking medication very regularly, but that is the easy way – just to remember to swallow a pill.

However, there are many far better and more effective ways to reduce the risk, but it takes dedication, commitment and effort – an effort to treat yourself kindly and to take responsibility for your illness.

What can we do to help ourselves?

The most effective treatments are:

• Stop smoking. Cigarette smoking is a potent risk factor for atherosclerosis. Statistics tell us that there is an increase of about 70 per cent in the death rate of smokers to non-smokers. The more cigarettes, cigars or pipe tobacco smoked and the longer you have smoked, the higher the incidence of dying from coronary artery disease

• Moderate your alcohol intake. Alcohol ingestion elevates serum cholesterol triglycerides and uric acid production, as well as increasing your blood pressure.

• Eat a sensible diet, free in the main from animal fats, additives, colourings and stimulants such as an excess of coffee, tea and caffeine drinks; colas in particular. Coffee in particular when drunk in an excess, and anything over 6 cups a day is excessive, increases the incidence of acute myocardial infarction.

• Do take a vitamin supplement. Garlic, lecithin, vitamin E and gingko biloba, all help the heart and the circulatory system. Yes, we do need supplements. The preparation of our food involves chemical sprays and synthetic manures in which our vegetables are grown and much of the vitamin content is lost before it even gets to our shops.

• Take some form of regular exercise: your heart is a strong pump. It likes to be used and it will become stronger if it is subjected to exercise on a regular basis.

Vitamins and minerals

I have mentioned the importance of vitamin and mineral supplementation and I shall now deal with the beneficial vitamins and minerals that will enhance the effectiveness of the circulatory system.

Vitamin B

Recent studies reveal that a deficiency in vitamin B is responsible for atherosclerosis in most individuals.

Vitamin E

A deficiency of this vitamin results in significantly higher levels of free radicals which cause increased damage, particularly of the vascular endothelium. Supplemental vitamin E has been shown to inhibit the platelet releasing action thus preventing the build up of atherosclerosis.

Vitamin C

High cholesterol levels can become elevated when there is a chronic low intake of vitamin C. This vitamin in particular helps fat metabolism and encourages the health of the arterial wall.

Magnesium

Magnesium offers significant protection against atherosclerosis as a deficiency of this mineral has been shown to produce spasms in the coronary arteries and is considered to be a cause of heart attacks in some cases – the spasms being the cause rather than a build up of plaque.

Magnesium assists in the strength of the contractions of the heart muscle. Not only has magnesium been found to be beneficial to those suffering from a heart attack but it is helpful in the management of irregular heart beat, particularly in the case of bradycardia and high blood pressure.

Although there is low incidence of cardiovascular disease in Greenland Eskimos, which has been linked to the high levels of EPA in their diet, high magnesium levels are a major part of the diet also, and encourages the low occurrence of heart disease.

Calcium carbonate

High cholesterol levels can also be reduced by the daily intake of 2 g of calcium carbonate.

Diet and recommended food factors for the treatment of coronary heart disease

Most authorities agree that the level of plasma cholesterol is largely determined by the dietary intake of total calories of cholesterol, polyunsaturated fat and saturated fat.

Vegetarian diet

Vegetarians have a much lower risk of developing heart disease. A vegetarian diet actually lowers the blood cholesterol levels. Cholesterol is produced by the liver and a fatty liver can triple its size, causing the common enormous bulge below the ribs in so many men to-day.

The liver cells become congested with fat, then cease to work effectively, which then puts a stress on every organ in the body. Remember that the body is a vibrating function: one system closely linked to another, creating a reciprocal arrangement. As a reflexologist you will undoubtedly find sensitivity in the liver reflex when treating patients with coronary heart disease.

Fibre

We hear much about the need for more fibre in our diet, and it is not just to make the digestive system perform its functions more effectively. Fibre sources which form a mucilaginous mass, and this will be found in pectin, oat bran and psyllium seed, bind bile and cholesterol in the intestines. They soak up the fat content and encourage fast elimination through the bowel.

Porridge in the mornings is such an excellent food, in aiding this function. A good, hearty, fried breakfast is just about the worst meal anybody suffering from heart conditions could ever indulge in, particularly as a start to the day.

Common sugar

This increases concentrations of plasma, cholesterol and uric acid, all of which are known to be involved in the development of atherosclerosis.

Fish oils (EPA)

A diet rich in fish oils often referred to as EPAs, which is common in many cold water fish – salmon, herring, and mackerel, to name but a few – should be eaten, at least three times a week.

Carnitine

A vitamin-like compound which initiates the breakdown of fatty acids; a decrease of this vitamin causes reduced energy production. If the heart does not have a good supply of oxygen, as would be the case in sufferers from angina or following a heart attack, the carnitine levels quickly decrease. Carnitine deficiency has been linked to diseases of the heart such as congestive heart failure and cardiac enlargement.

Onions and garlic

Onions have been proved to counteract the increased platelet aggregation seen after consumption of a high fat meal and have been shown to have anti-hypertensive and cholesterol lowering effects. Garlic has similar effects, but it also thins the blood, thus aiding better flow through the arteries.

Diet and lifestyle

There is absolutely no doubt that atherosclerosis is a disease of affluence, not poverty, and eliminating all known risk factors as discussed above requires major changes in diet, and lifestyle to be maintained by the patient on a permanent basis.

Increase the intake of vegetables and fruits: dietary fibre is essential. Cold pressed vegetable oils, fish oil and olive oil are excellent. Reduce the consumption of saturated fats. Throw your frying pan away and take ginger, garlic and onions daily.

The individual with angina should stop smoking and take only moderate amounts of alcohol, one or two glasses of red or white wine a day is the maximum.

Everytime you drink a cup of coffee, particularly if it is strong and black with white sugar, it is just like putting your foot on the accelerator of the car: adrenalin is released, the body is geared up and heart rate and blood pressure rise.

Just imagine the stress on the heart if you are putting it through this stress eight or nine times a day – rather like slow suicide!

Learn to relax. Maybe one of those guided imagery tapes will help you to let every part of your body become limp and peaceful.

Walking is the best exercise, but you do need to walk briskly so that you are aware of your heart beating and begin to perspire, this ensures that the blood is pulsating forcefully through the body. Aerobic exercises and swimming are highly recommended.

To reiterate, you would be advised to take a multivitamin tablet daily and Vitamin E, 200 iu per day. A fibre supplement such as psyllium seed, 5 g daily, is excellent. Vitamin C, 2g per day. Olive oil or linseed oil, 1-2 tblsp a day and EPA, 10g per day.

The main areas to treat with reflexology

When treating your patient or loved one who is suffering from any of the diseases of propulsion, and that includes, angina, coronary heart disease, atherosclerosis, hypertension and low blood pressure, the main areas to treat are as shown in the following diagrams.

It is perfectly safe to treat the patient on a daily basis if you have the opportunity so to do. *See Figures 30.1, 30.2 and 30.3.*

Working the heart

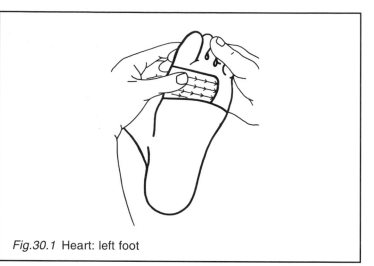

Fig.30.1 Heart: left foot

Working the thoracic spine

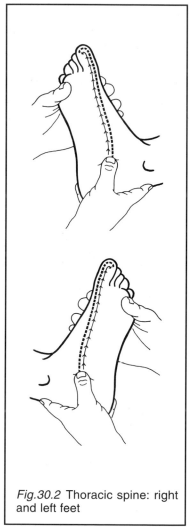

Fig.30.2 Thoracic spine: right and left feet

Working the lungs

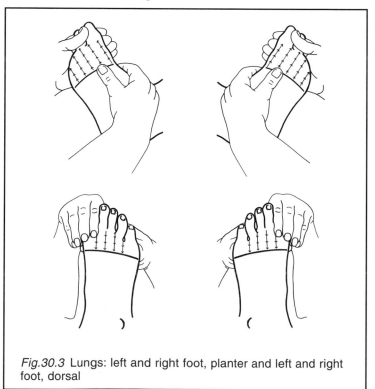

Fig.30.3 Lungs: left and right foot, planter and left and right foot, dorsal

CHAPTER 31 Reflexology for babies

Babies enjoy the relaxing effect of reflexology just as much as other people do.

The working out of the reflexes in a baby's foot is simple as you will notice that, until they are about four or five, there is little arch on the underside of the foot. In fact, a baby's foot really resembles an oval. *See Figure 31.1.*

It is because of the shape of a baby's foot that we just need to cover the complete surface of the foot, starting at the heel and working up the entire area to the join of the toes with the foot, using tiny, forward-creeping movements.

Another all important area to work is the inside of both feet which resembles the spine, right up to the top of the big toe which, you will remember, is the area to the brain.

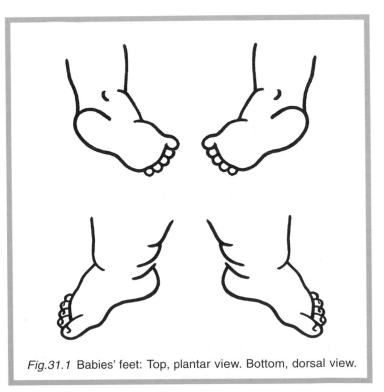

Fig.31.1 Babies' feet: Top, plantar view. Bottom, dorsal view.

THE BENEFITS OF REFLEXOLOGY

1 Birth traumas

The spinal area is of major benefit to those babies who suffered a traumatic birth, such as a prolonged labour which may result in a forceps delivery.

Frequently incessant crying, or difficulties in establishing good feeding habits, can be the result of a hazardous journey into the world for, although the birth canal is relatively short, our exit from the uterus into the outside world can be the most hazardous journey we ever make.

2 Colic

Apart from birth traumas, another distressing condition which affects many babies in the first three months of life is colic, particularly evening colic when, between the hours of seven and ten, the baby cries and seems to be full of wind, and the more the crying continues the more air is taken into the digestive system and so a vicious circle begins.

Try working on the entire surface of the baby's feet during these restless periods. Reflexology will certainly help the digestive system and ease the painful episodes of wind and pain.

ALLERGY AND DIET

Allergy is not an illness, it is a symptom of a condition and an indication that something is wrong. We need symptoms in order to take some action to do something about them.

1 Infantile eczema

Babies can be born with an allergic reaction to foods and have outbreaks of eczema, which is both unsightly and very distressing to the baby, as well as the mother.

Sometimes the very food that the mother craved for during pregnancy was the food that, because it was eaten or drunk in excess, caused the allergic reaction in the baby.

Some mothers have a desire for fizzy drinks and there are frequently artificial sweeteners in these drinks which many have an allergy to. Others have a need for chocolate: there are many artificial colourings in chocolate that can also have an effect. The list of allergens is endless.

Keep the baby's skin well oiled with a light olive oil, rather than using medicated creams.

2 Cradle cap

Cradle cap is another sign of possible allergy, so eczema should be regarded as a danger signal from the body that certain foods are causing a stress on the baby's delicate digestive system.

3 Breast feeding and allergy

Breast feeding is always best. Not only does breast feeding help to build a strong digestive and immune system, but there is now evidence to suppose that long term breast feeding actually helps to prevent cancer.

The mother should make absolutely sure that her diet is as natural as possible: a vegetarian diet is preferable if you have a baby suffering from eczema – there are few vegetables, fruits and pulses that cause an allergy. Plenty of carbohydrates in the form of rices, pasta, wheatmeal bread, potatoes, and a good intake of calcium in the form of a tablet when you are breast feeding is preferable to drinking large quantities of milk and eating cheese, as your baby may well be allergic to dairy products.

Make sure that the fluid intake is sufficient. Drink juices, preferably apple, grape and mango. Orange juice can be the cause of allergic reactions. Remember, it is not necessary to drink lots of milk to produce breast milk. It *is* necessary to drink a lot of fluid.

4 Weaning

When it comes to weaning the baby, follow the same dietary rules as above and do not introduce any foods from the cow until the baby has his first grinding teeth which will be towards the end of the second year. You can be sure that by this time the digestive system will have become mature and there will be far less likelihood of an allergic skin reaction.

CHAPTER **32**   The spinal connection

The central nervous system conveys messages from that magical computer – our brain. We have 12 pairs of nerves arising from the brain and 31 pairs of nerves directing their powerful influence to all parts of the human body. *See Figure 32.1.*

If you could, therefore, just work with the very fine balance of tiny, creeping forward movements on the inside of the feet, which is the contact area for the spinal nerves, you would be helping the entire bodily functions. *See Figures 32.2, 32.3 and Chapter 17.*

The Spinal Chart in this chapter, *see Figure 32.4,* will show you how, by stimulating a specific area in the spinal reflexes, you will be able to help conditions in the body. This reference showing the application of working specific parts of the spinal area for specific parts of the human body should not be studied or practised until you are well qualified as a reflexology practitioner and have some experience. You can then branch out further into working just a small refined area in the spine to assist a particular organ or function.

As you gain confidence and experience in your work as a reflexologist, you will be able to refer back to the spinal chart and concentrate your efforts in working that part of the spinal cord which will give aid and support to the appropriate part of the body that is congested, out of balance or tense.

You need to isolate that tiny, pinprick point in the spinal area with your index finger and when found, work on the reflex point with rotating movements with your mid finger when working from the lumbar to the thoracic areas, and then the index finger to work out the area to the cervical spine, following the diagrams to find the correct procedures to adopt when working out these areas.

Always remember that 'Structure Governs Function' and any imbalance or compression of a nerve pathway affects the ultimate functioning of any organ, gland or part of the human body.

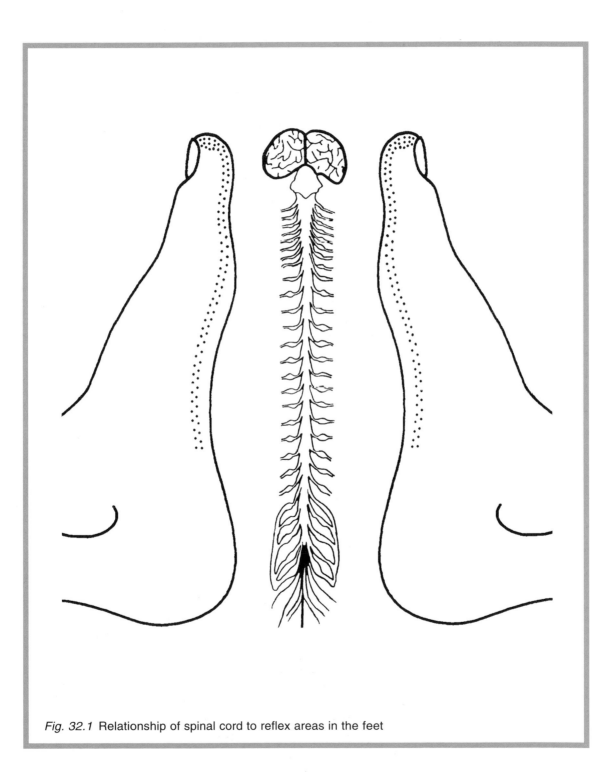

Fig. 32.1 Relationship of spinal cord to reflex areas in the feet

Working the lumbar and thoracic spine

These diagrams show the support for working the lumbar and thoracic spine.

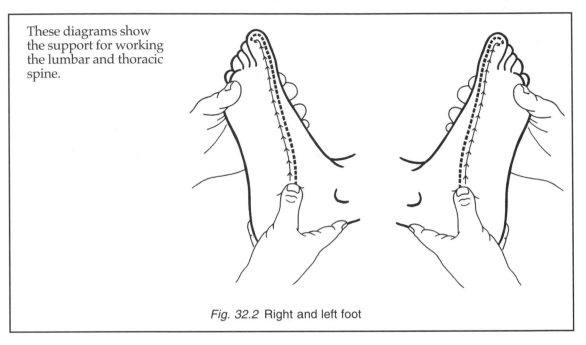

Fig. 32.2 Right and left foot

Working the cervical spine

These diagrams show the support for working out the cervical spine.

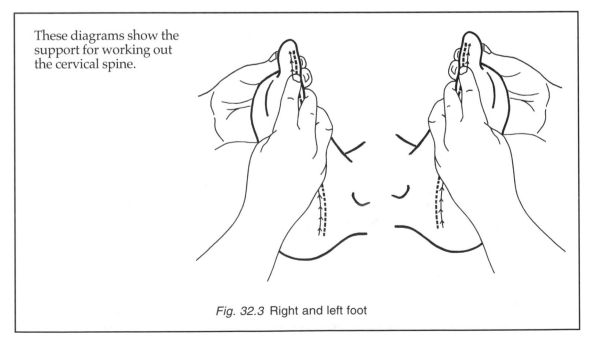

Fig. 32.3 Right and left foot

Spinal chart

1 - 7 **Cervical**	**CERVICAL 1**	Blood supply to the cranium, pituitary, hypothalamus, pineal, inner and middle ear
	CERVICAL 2	The eyes, sinuses, forehead, mouth
	CERVICAL 3	Trigeminal nerve, outer ear, teeth
	CERVICAL 4	The nasal passages, eustachian tube
	CERVICAL 5	Pharynx, larynx
1 - 12 **Thoracic**	**CERVICAL 6**	Shoulders and neck muscles
	CERVICAL 7	The thyroid gland, shoulders, elbows
	THORACIC 1–5	The head, neck and heart
	THORACIC 2–4	Bronchi and lung
	THORACIC 2–5	The upper limbs
	THORACIC 5–6	Oesophagus
	THORACIC 6–10	Stomach
	THORACIC 7–9	Liver and gall bladder
	THORACIC 9–10	Small intestine
1 - 5 **Lumbar**	**THORACIC 10-L2**	Lower limbs
	THORACIC 11–L1	Large intestine as far as splenic flexure
	THORACIC 10–L1	Kidney and Fallopian tubes
	THORACIC 11–L2	Ureter
	THORACIC 8–L1	Suparenal
	THORACIC 10–11	Testis and ovary
	THORACIC 11–12	Epididymis, vas deferens, seminal vesicles
	THORACIC 11–L2	Urinary bladder
Sacrum 5 fused bones	**THORACIC 11–L1**	Prostate and prostatic urethra
	THORACIC 12–L1	Uterus
	LUMBAR 1–2	Splenic flexure to rectum
Coccyx 4 fused bones		*Fig. 32.4* Spinal chart

CHAPTER **33**   Drug reactions

It is essential to have an understanding of the side effects of a variety of drugs that are used in controlling symptoms and pain in various conditions.

Shortly after I started in my practice some 25 years ago, I frequently found a sensitivity in the foot which did not really seem to relate to the condition that I was treating.

As an example, I would be treating a patient with severe hay fever and would pick up a sensitivity in the sinus and lung areas in the foot which I expected, but I would then find that the kidney area was extremely sensitive.

This was confusing. What on earth had the kidneys to do with hay fever? As the months went by there would be more and more queries.

Sensitivities appeared in the feet which just did not link up to the problem the patient had come to me with. Maybe the chart I was using was incorrect, or was there some other hidden mystery concerning reflexology that I knew nothing about? Perhaps I would have to try and work this out for myself?

I noted that patients presenting with these various odd sensitivities were all on medications of some kind or another

Eventually, after consulting an encyclopaedia of drugs, I realised that what I was in fact picking up were the congested areas in the body caused by the medications that the patients were taking.

Drugs and how they affect the reflexes
As we all know, drugs have side effects and cause inflammation and congestion and upset the functioning of other parts of the body.

The following list describes some everyday groups of drugs and the effects they have on the body, and the sensitivities they create in the reflexes to the organs, to be found in the feet.

DRUGS AND THEIR REACTIONS

Anti-histamine Commonly used for allergic reactive illnesses, e.g. hay fever, skin rashes, troublesome irritant coughs and eczema. Anti-histamines create an inflammation in the kidney reflex area of the foot.

Steroids Frequently used to break down inflammation and therefore commonly used for arthritis, heart conditions, cancer and severe allergic reactive illness such as asthma, which has become out of control. Taking steroids can create an insensitivity in the foot; therefore you are likely to find no reaction at all, but it is worth while giving treatment as it still has a beneficial effect upon the body. Steroids lower a person's vitality.

Nonsteroidal anti-inflammatory drugs Used in the control of arthritis and rheumatism, gout and inflammatory conditions of the spine.

Aspirin Commonly used to kill pain. Creates stomach inflammation and sometimes stomach ulceration. Many people are allergic to aspirin.

Painkillers All painkilling drugs have a disastrous effect on the intestine and normally cause chronic constipation.

Antibiotics Commonly used to control infections in the body. They destroy the flora content in the intestine which upsets the balance of the body and can either cause constipation or diarrhoea. The liver is always affected when these drugs are used.

Antidepressant drugs/sleeping pills These types of medication cause great sensitivity in the brain area of the foot.

Beta-blockers Used in the control of heart conditions and hypertension. They dull the sensitivity of the body and thus work as a depressant to the adrenal gland and the heart causing the heart beat to become slower. They also have an effect upon the liver.

Amphetamines These drugs are used in an attempt to reduce appetite for weight control. They are extremely addictive and stimulate all functioning of the body to work overtime thereby creating a drastic effect on the central nervous system. The brain and adrenal glands are usually acutely sensitive in those taking this drug.

Antacids Medications for digestive disturbances: peppermint flavoured and chalk based. The chalk content in this type of medication has an effect upon the kidneys and can cause kidney stones if taken in large quantities over a long period of time.

CHAPTER **34**   Areas of assistance

An area of assistance is an area or system of the body that is instrumental in helping to remedy dysfunctions in other parts, even though the area in question may seem to have no particular relationship to the illness. Frequently the assisted area is in the same zone, details and examples of which are shown below.

Condition	Assisted area	Why?
Shoulder conditions	*The hip area*	Because it is in the same zone and creates a balancing effect on the structure of the body.
Hip conditions	*The shoulder*	The same.
Asthma and all allergic and respiratory conditions, including eczema	*The digestive system and adrenals*	Allergy usually starts in the digestive system in infancy. Also the lung and digestive systems are in the same five zones.
Knee conditions	*Lumbar spine*	Most knee conditions other than specific troubles such as arthritis in the knee or knee injuries are caused by compression of the lumbar spinal nerves.
Eye and ear conditions	*Kidney and cervical spine*	Because it is in the same zone and medically it is accepted that the eyes are affected when there are dysfunctions in the kidney.
Infertility (if a hormonal imbalance)	*Endocrine*	Irregular cycles are often caused by hormonal imbalances.
Infertility (from organic causes)	*The reproductive system*	Could have nothing to do with the hormonal system.

Condition	Assisted area	Why?
Pains in the calf	*Lumbar spine and entire circulatory system*	Could be spinal compression in the lumbar area or a circulatory problem in the legs. It is a common symptom in diabetics and in those suffering from arteriosclerosis when the heart is under strain and is unable to pump the blood efficiently to the extremities, i.e. the legs. This condition is commonly known as intermittent claudication.
Weakness in the hands and tingling in the fingers	*The cervical spine*	Compression in the neck
Any underactive condition such as an underactive thyroid	*Work on pituitary and adrenal glands to stimulate body.*	To encourage some extra activity in the thyroid.
Any overactive condition	*Work on the solar plexus to calm and avoid the adrenal glands.*	To bring about a calming and relaxed effect in the body.
Vertigo (dizziness)	*Often helps to work on the cervical spine.*	Improves nerve and blood supply to the head.
Lumps and cysts in the breast	*The endocrine system*	Frequently caused by an endocrine imbalance.
Palpitations (racing heart)	*Often the stomach area*	Unless there is a known heart condition, indigestion can cause pressure from the stomach on the heart and can create these symptoms.

Condition	Assisted area	Why?
Depression	*The endocrine system*	Often a hormonal imbalance.
Exhaustion	*Thyroid and adrenal glands*	Helps stimulate the body.
Heart conditions	*Liver and thoracic spine*	The liver has a responsibility in the circulatory system; controls the clotting factor, produces the cholesterol levels. Spinal nerves in the thoracic spine help heart muscle function.
Constipation	*Liver and lumbar spine*	Gall lubricates the bowel and the lumbar spinal nerves stimulate nerve function to the pelvic area.
Indigestion	*Liver and thoracic spine*	Thoracic spinal nerves improve blood supply to the liver.
Migraine	*Liver and cervical spine*	Helps detoxification and relaxes tension in the neck.
Fluid retention in the legs	*All the main lymphatic areas plus urinary system*	To help balance the fluid levels and help elimination.
Varicose veins	*Intestines and lumbar spine*	Any pressure in the intestinal area, i.e. constipation, a prolapsed condition of the bowel which is often found in those suffering from colitis, and diverticulitis can cause varicose conditions of the legs. Working on the lumbar spine can improve the nerve and blood supply to the entire pelvic areas.

CHAPTER **35** # The do's and don'ts of reflexology

Do not offer a cure. Professing to be able to 'cure' anything is rather a bold statement. The aim of the reflexology practitioner is to be able to relieve pain, improve bodily functions and assist in aiding the body to eliminate its waste more efficiently, particularly through the liver which becomes very congested today with all the chemicals and toxins which pollute our planet thus creating stress on the organs of elimination.

'Curing' really means restoring the body to a near perfect state permanently. There is no treatment anywhere, whether in the orthodox or complementary medical fields that can offer this.

Many people are relieved of their disturbing symptoms and attend for an occasional treatment – say, every six weeks – and find that this 'maintenance treatment' keeps them in tip-top condition for years and years. Other patients prefer to have their treatment sessions, gain the maximum possible improvement in their health and then stop treatment altogether and just see how their health continues. It is not unusual for patients to return to their original practitioner after a seven year gap.

Patients always return to where they received the greatest benefit in their health.

1 Is it possible to give a course of reflexology treatments?

Generally speaking, the average person responds very well in six sessions conducted on a weekly basis. Some people take longer and in most instances the chronic states take a little longer to improve than acute problems.

The best way is to give your treatment sessions weekly until the patients remarks that their pains or symptoms have greatly improved; at that stage lengthen the appointment gap to fortnightly. If a good result has been maintained over a fortnightly session, then it is totally safe to leave the gap this time for a month. After the month's gap, if all symptoms and pain levels have failed to return, it is a very good indication that a good result has been achieved with reflexology. It is then up to the patient to decide whether they wish to return once every six weeks for a general 'maintenance treatment' or cease reflexology treatments altogether and just see what happens.

2 Do keep all information strictly confidential

To keep good records of your patients is essential. It is also essential to make sure that information which they give you will be in the strictest confidence.

I will deal with necessary information that should be included in record keeping in Chapter 37, The Treatment Session.

3 Don't change your techniques

There is never any need to change the practical reflexology techniques which you have been trained to use at **The British School of Reflexology**. The techniques of reflexology are superb and work beautifully without any changes needing to be made. I have been using the same techniques now for 25 years and the achievements obtained in such a variety of chronic and acute medical conditions still never fail to surprise and delight me.

It is not possible to be a practitioner of reflexology, or any other science which involves treating sick people, if you know little or nothing about the causes of disease and dysfunction. It is, therefore, practical and sensible to attend the further training courses offered at your School where you can extend your knowledge of illness and the treatment of disease. Patients feel very safe in the hands of a practitioner who is not only proficient and professional at their skill but is also able to communicate with patients in an informed manner on their own particular illness or disease.

It gives a secure feeling to the patient when the rapport between the therapist and themselves is such that they feel confident that the reflexologist's knowledge is extensive enough for their symptoms and conditions to be understood.

So read more about the body, mind and spirit; go to as many workshops and lectures as you possibly can; enjoy soaking up information remembering that **knowledge instills confidence**!

4 How much pressure is needed for reflexology to be effective?

Sufficient pressure should be applied to be totally acceptable to the patient without causing them any undue distress or for them to feel the need to withdraw their feet from your hands. For the patient to do so would indicate a very poor reflexology treatment. It does not 'take a sledgehammer to crack a nut' and as long as the pressure is consistent and applied in a professional manner, which is enjoyable for the patient, this is a good guide to its efficacy and the expertise needed.

I usually ask my patients, 'Is this pressure sufficient for you or am I able to go into the foot with a deeper pressure?' Obviously, it is the patient who is receiving the treatment and you must be guided by what is acceptable to them.

You will need to use a much firmer pressure when treating, for example, the size 11 foot of a tall strong man than for the small foot of a child of five. This is just common sense. It is pointless working over anybody's foot with a 'feather touch technique'. It is necessary to really get into the reflex point, so there is need for a firm consistent pressure with the thumb and a comfortable support for the foot at all times.

5 No additional aids

Reflexology is such a simple treatment because you do not need any additional aids. All that you *do* need are two hands, which will be trained to work in a precise and professional way, and knowledge, which can be gained from the professional training courses – and obviously, a patient to whom we can apply our expertise. No oils, creams, lotions, or probes, or any form of electrical stimulating devices are necessary to give a good reflexology treatment. It is a 'hands-on' treatment with a total one-to-one communication between patient and therapist during the whole course of the treatment session.

6 Patients with infectious illnesses

It is inadvisable to treat a patient during the acute stage of an infectious illness. Reflexology is a stimulating science and tends to create a detoxifying effect on all the eliminating functions of the body: the lungs, kidneys, bowels, sinuses and skin. During an acute infection, the body is desperately trying to rid itself of an accumulation of toxins.

Disease manifests itself when within 24 hours the body fails to eliminate all its waste matter efficiently. The excess of toxic waste eventually reaches a dangerously high level, the body is becoming overloaded with waste and, as a safety valve, your life energy produces a cold; your influenza attack; your stomach upset which causes diahorrea and/or vomiting. These are all ways of eliminating waste, even if in a rather aggressive fashion!

If we work, therefore, on those eliminating functions of the body during any acute infectious attack, we are just encouraging the body to eliminate even more toxins and this will make the patient feel even more disturbed and unwell than before.

By all means work on the reflexes to the pituitary gland in cases of high temperature – this has a good result in lowering temperature. Work on the relaxation techniques to create a feeling of relaxation in the patient, but do avoid those organs of elimination at the acute stage of an infectious illness. It is best to begin treating the patient after they have recovered from their illness, in the 'passive' stage.

7 Patients with long term health problems

I always suggest, when treating patients who have had a long term history of frequent medication and perhaps are in rather poor health, that the reflexologist under-treats on the first occasion. Use a very light pressure, do not exceed half an hour of working over the feet, and just wait for a report from the patient as to how they felt the day after their treatment session.

You might ask whether they felt that their condition had worsened; if they had any bowel or bladder problems; whether they were suffering from a severe headache; etcetera. Be guided by these reactions. In the case of an elderly person who suffers extreme reaction to a treatment session, they may not feel confident in returning for a further appointment.

If all is well after the initial treatment and the patient reports a general feeling of improvement and well being, then it is quite in order to increase the duration of the treatment session and perhaps use a slightly more intense pressure.

Remember, the patient is your guide.

8 Can reflexology be dangerous?

There are no dangers attached to reflexology, as we are only treating a reflex point in the foot that links to a corresponding part of the body.

We are not applying any undue pressure or manipulation on the body as would happen in the case of an osteopathic treatment. We are not giving the patient any medications to ingest into the system. We are not putting any oils or lotions on to the feet which could perhaps affect skin tone.

The greatest benefit that we can achieve with reflexology is total relaxation and, as stress is the cause of most disease, we are well on the way to defeating a host of illnesses that people suffer by eliminating emotional stresses which affect the functions of the body.

I have treated patients suffering from strokes and heart conditions, pregnant women and brain damaged children, to name but a few, and have had some outstanding results in all aspects of health.

There are some circumstances where I would use extreme care, and they would simply be for the diabetic who has very frail skin tone on their feet with perhaps poor circulation. I would not treat diabetics if they had any breaks in the skin area such as an ulcer on the foot or something of this nature. It would be best to wait until these problems had been healed by appropriate medical treatment or use hand reflexology.

It is quite safe to treat pregnant women. Pregnancy is a natural function, not an illness, and most women find that reflexology is of tremendous assistance in helping to prevent fluid retention which causes feet and hands to swell and be uncomfortable; to keep their blood pressure normal and to avoid distressing episodes of back pain.

There would be just one circumstance where I would refrain from giving treatment in pregnancy and that would be when a patient coming to me had a history of frequent miscarriage, say, at 12 to 14 weeks. I would be much happier to wait until this period of time had elapsed as, when a miscarriage does occur, patients go through a period of grief and normally look to blame somebody for the miscarriage, and it would be very unfortunate if reflexology were to be linked to the cause of their miscarriage.

If patients suffer conditions such as a verrucae or a corn, it is quite safe to give treatment providing the verrucae is covered with a sticking plaster.

Postoperatively, reflexology is helpful as the shock and distress associated with surgery is something, which I feel, reflexology is very effective in countering.

Surgery also has a very debilitating effect on the immune system, and again reflexology can be of benefit in restoring the immune system in the body.

9 Is it safe to give reflexology treatments daily?

It is totally safe to treat patients daily, although it is unlikely that the average person will be able to attend for a daily session for practical and financial reasons. However, a member of your family or a friend will be able to enjoy a daily treatment session and it is particularly beneficial when treating acute back conditions such as sciatica, lumbago, disc lesions and so on. It is also beneficial to treat asthmatic sufferers every day in order to try and relax their lungs and heart function and to benefit their general health.

10 Can I treat the very elderly and the very young?

It is totally safe to treat everyone, regardless of age. I have treated infants under a year old and my oldest patient was 99 years old.

11 Do I need to get permission from a medical doctor before commencing treatment?

There is absolutely no need to get permission from the doctor or anybody else involved in the medical profession before commencing treatment with the very safe and effective methods of reflexology.

Always remember that your body is your total responsibility, it does not belong to the doctor, and we all have the right to choose exactly how we wish our bodies to be treated, just as we choose which foods to eat, which car we drive, which hair style suits us best and the colour of our clothes.

Most people have tried reflexology treatments when all else has failed. They have consulted their doctors, taken drugs, and maybe have had surgery, and still their condition prevails. They find that reflexology is an acceptable treatment and one which they feel gives them maximum support.

12 Be realistic in your aims

If you are a practitoner of reflexology, treating patients regularly, you will need to decide for yourself what are your specific aims and the relief that you expect to be able to achieve with patients suffering a variety of conditions.

It must be obvious to you that if you are treating a patient who has been confined to a wheelchair for many years suffering from multiple sclerosis and maybe has acute and frequent bladder infections, then your talents and the relief which you would be able to offer the patient would be minimal. I expect that the main help you could offer would be to improve their general circulation and perhaps to reduce the number of bladder infections and generally give them a feeling of well-being, thus improving their quality of life. There is no way in which a person who has been chair-bound for this length of time would be able to restore movement or walk again.

Similarly, with a patient who had a long history of asthma and was now middle-aged and who for most of their life had been treated with inhalers of a steroidal nature in order for them to be able to main some quality of life, the results which you would expect to achieve would be a reduction in the number of attacks suffered with less severity. It would be very doubtful whether such a patient would be able to be restored to full health and strength as, generally speaking, long term sufferers from asthma have quite a lot of impairment of lung function and often an enlarged heart due to the excessive strain which the heart has been under for years in coping with a limited oxygen supply during the times of acute asthma attacks.

There again, if you were treating a young man who maybe had a back strain caused by the heavy physical work which he had undertaken, the achievements that you could anticipate would be total relief.

You must therefore take a realistic approach to the treatment of patients and understand that, although reflexology is a wonderfully beneficial treatment for a host of physical conditions, it is not the panacea to all the illnesses of mankind.

13 Can I treat cancer?

Many books written on reflexology warn people off the treatment for cancer sufferers. I have treated cancer patients for years, and with only good results, and although reflexology can in no way cure cancer, nor can profess to be able to stop secondaries appearing, I have found generally speaking that patients have all exclaimed how much better they have felt. They experienced a great sense of relief and I think in the main a freedom from anxiety. Medical doctors and researchers agree the increase in stress and the pace of living over the last 50 years or so, plus the introduction of the western fast food diet have made a great contribution to the increase in cancer. Surely then, as reflexology is of admirable support in creating relaxation to the body, mind and spirit, it must be a benefit in this condition.

Many practitioners are working in hospices throughout the country. Their presence is greatly respected by the medical profession. Patients enjoy the treatment sessions and ask for a return visit, and, after all, if a patient only has a very short time to live then it really is up to the patient to decide for themselves if reflexology gives them relief and a feeling of wellbeing.

The relatives of the terminally ill patient also find it rewarding to have been able to offer something to their suffering relative, and I think perhaps it saves any 'guilt complex' after the death of a loved one to feel that they did in fact respect any request for care which the patient asked for.

More detailed information is to be found in Chapter 29 on the facts and support for those suffering from cancer.

14 Areas of assistance

Reflexology is not just about treating the part of the body that hurts by means of the relative part of the foot. There is a great understanding of how root causes for illness are often created in another area frequently far from the ailing part.

15 Pain control

It is vital that reflexologists have a good insight into the role that they are to play in the relief of pain in the care of sick people and the benefits that are likely to be obtained with reflexology.

Generally speaking most of the everyday conditions which one would take to the GP can be greatly relieved, and in many cases the symptoms removed altogether, by frequent treatments of reflexology by a well qualified practitioner.

16 We do not diagnose, prescribe or profess to 'cure'

There has been much confusion regarding 'diagnosis'. Reflexology is not able to diagnose diseases within the body. However, what the practitioner can find is that a corresponding part of the foot will reveal a great sensitivity and this in turn indicates that there is congestion, inflammation and tension in that part of the body. Frequently, by treating the sensitive areas, the inflammation is relieved, tension removed and great improvement in the functioning of the system of the body that is under duress is achieved.

When a sensitivity is found in the foot, it is absolutely wrong for the practitioner to jump to the conclusion that 'if Mrs. Smith's liver reflex points reveal a great sensitivity' then, surely, she must be suffering from a liver disease. This is diagnosing, particularly if the reflexologist adds medical terms to the sensitivity found in the foot – 'I think perhaps this patient is suffering from hepatitis or cirrhosis of the liver.'

A sensitivity in the liver can be due to many factors. It could be due to an over-indulgence of alcohol in the days before a treatment session. It could be due to an indulgence in a meal with a heavy fat content which burdens the liver's ability to eliminate.

It could also indicate a high cholesterol level, and if you were treating a patient with angina, or coronary artery disease, this could well be the cause of the sensitivity. Remember that the fat content of the blood is dealt with by the liver; cholesterol is formed here.

Nevertheless, the practitioner is in no way able to diagnose these precise problems. Only doctors are able to diagnose disease for they have access to X-ray machines, equipment for blood tests, scanning devices and so on.

Similar situations can occur when a reflexology practitioner picks up a great sensitivity in the heart reflex area. Remember that, although the heart is a muscular area, the position of the heart reflex points within the foot also link up to the muscles within the chest (such as the pectoral muscles). These can easily become over-strained by an episode of heavy lifting, gardening or even perhaps carrying a toddler on one side for too long a period. The muscles then become over-strained and, when the foot is worked upon, show up great sensitivities in the chest and heart area.

It is completely unprofessional for any practitioner to jump to the conclusion that this person now has a 'heart condition' and it would be totally wrong

and unethical for them to make such suggestions.

Reflexologists are reflexologists and doctors are doctors, and we cannot mix the two together but there is no reason at all why in the future, reflexologists should not work alongside the medical profession.

We must always respect the many years of study that doctors have had in the treatment and care of patients, whereas the practitioner of reflexology, in the main, has had a very short course, which certainly does not entitle them to diagnose illness.

17 Aims and objectives

It is necessary to assess the situation which is before you and produce a realistic picture of the amount of relief you are going to be able to give your patients.

Reflexology can help in nearly all cases. In fact, we find through our long years of experience in treating people with all manner of illness, that only about six per cent of people fail to respond to reflexology treatment.

There is no real reason why these people do not get the improvement which was expected. It can often be some simple condition which you have treated many times before but find in this instance that the patient simply does not respond.

Conversely, there could be some very complicated long term illness which suddenly responds dramatically to reflexology after just one or two treatment sessions. There really is no rhyme or reason why these oddities occur.

Generally speaking people who have attended treatment for at least six weekly sessions do get good results. There are very few people who attend for that period of time who can honestly say at the end of the course of treatments that reflexology has done absolutely nothing for them whatsoever.

However, as nothing works for everybody, we must accept that there will be that very small percentage who just do not respond to reflexology. I then advise these patients to try some other form of complementary medicine, such as acupuncture, herbalism or something similar.

18 Side effects following reflexology treatment

It is not unusual to get side effects following a treatment of reflexology. It is essential therefore that the patient and the practitioner are well aware of exactly what is going on within the body when these symptoms occur.

Symptoms are signals of changes in the body and following a treatment it is not unusual for the patient to discover that her symptoms have become exacerbated; her back pain may be worse; and there may be a frequency of bowel actions or an increase in the output of urine. Sinuses may begin to stream and, if the patient suffers from a chest infection, there may be large quantities of mucus coughed up from the lungs.

These are all excellent signs of a healing crisis – proof enough, that reflexology works.

Reflexology is a stimulating science. It aims to improve circulation and helps the body rid itself of unwanted substances. Any build-up or residue of toxins causes a 'stagnation' in one or other vital areas and this in turn leads to congestion.

As we use reflexology we create a stimulating effect on the organic functions of the body which can express itself in a temporary worsening of symptoms. The same symptoms occur when having treatment with herbal preparations, homoeopathic support, fasts and colonic irrigations.

I must make it quite clear that this in no way means that the patient has 'become worse'. This is a true indication of a 'healing crisis' and would be a welcomed sign by any practitioner working within the naturopathic field of healing.

I have even known patients come out in a rash following a treatment session and as the skin is a great organ of elimination, this again is a healing sign, and a way in which the body can rid itself of toxins.

One very positive result following a treatment session is that the patient makes a claim that they slept for many hours following the session, or that their general sleep pattern improved. This is a total breakdown in the stress of the body, creating within the patient a feeling of harmony and relief.

Nature needs a clean slate upon which to build her foundation of health. When we take medication for a condition we are simply embedding the problem deeper within the body, and from time to time we will experience another set of symptoms as the problems within the body 'burst through' and express themselves in yet another form.

It is impossible to suppress nature; she will always have her revenge in yet another part or system of the body. When treating with complementary medicines, particularly reflexology, we are treating the root cause of disease and trying to restore the balance and harmony, improve nerve and blood supply and help the body to detoxify itself in an improved form. Once this cleansing and relaxation has occurred, then the body is in the right condition to heal itself.

There are no dangers in treating with reflexology and it is impossible to make a situation within the body permanently worse.

Advice to offer to your patients following a treatment session, particularly if the problem is of an organic nature, say irritable bowel syndrome, arthritis, asthma, migraine, sinusitis, would be for them to drink a large quantity of pure, bottled spring water and take a large dose of vitamin C: 1g would not be too much on this occasion. Vitamin C helps detoxification and the extra fluids help flush the toxic waste through the urinary system. This will lessen the possible side effects of the treatment.

It is unusual to continue having side effects with reflexology after the first couple of treatments. Thereafter all should be plain sailing, and the patient should find that their condition improves little by little, week by week

until, at the end of between six and eight sessions, they should have an excellent result from their particular health problem.

The introduction of regular reflexology treatments gives great relief from both mental and physical stress and patients become aware of a new feeling of well-being which has perhaps been foreign to them until now. This is the greatest asset that this wonderful treatment can provide.

Conclusion

The professional support and advice offered in this book will give you, the practitioner, a guide to the development of your practice and skill as a professional reflexologist. However, reflexology can never be learnt from just purchasing a book and looking at a colourful chart. You do need the training of an expert who has been involved in the field of reflexology as a practitioner in treating patients, and as a teacher involved in the training of practitioners throughout the world.

I have shared with you in this book my experiences of reflexology and the practical application of reflexology shown here should make it easy for you as a practitioner to work on a patient and make the treatment session enjoyable for the patient receiving it.

Reflexology still proves to be a very safe and effective way of helping people. The only instruments we need to support our work are two well-trained hands, the professional knowledge which you will gain from our training courses, and the desire and compassion to help people

CHAPTER **36** Reference guide to treating specific conditions

Condition	Symptoms	Main area to treat
Addison's disease	*Adrenal insufficiency.*	Whole of the endocrine system.
Alzheimer's disease	*Degeneration of cerebral cortex. Loss of memory and paralysis.*	Extensive work on whole of spine and brain, preferably daily.
Ankylosing spondylitis	*Disease of joints, destruction of joint space followed by sclerosis and calcification, resulting in rigidity of spinal column and thorax.*	Spine, brain, shoulder, hip, knee, coccyx and pelvis. Adrenals to help break down inflammation.
Arteritis	*Inflammation of arteries.*	Heart/lung, thoracic spine, adrenals.
Bronchitis and asthma	*Inflammation of bronchial tubes. Spasm of the bronchioles, resulting in difficulty in exhalation.*	Heart/lung, adrenals, thoracic spine (to help nerve supply to thoracic area), digestive system (often a weakness in the digestive system causes excessive mucus in the system.
Bursitis	*Inflammation of a bursa.*	Work the relative joint, e.g. knee/elbow, plus lumbar spine in the case of knee: cervical spine for elbow. Helps the nerve supply to the affected part.
Cancer	*Depends on the organ involved.*	The whole of the body, especially the spleen to help the immune system.

Condition	Symptoms	Main area to treat
Candida	*A fungus causing thrush.*	The whole of the intestinal and reproductive area.
Carpal tunnel syndrome	*Numbness and tingling in the fingers and hands: the result of compression of median nerve of the wrist.*	Cervical spine and elbow area to aid nerve supply to the wrist.
Cataract	*Opacity of lens of eye.*	Eye, sinuses, cervical spine.
Cerebral haemorrhage (stroke)	*Rupture of an artery of the brain due to either high blood pressure or disease of artery.*	Entire spine, brain, respiratory, circulatory and kidney (to help renal blood supply and, ultimately, blood pressure).
Cerebral palsy (spasticity)	*Condition in which the control of the motor system is affected due to a lesion resulting from a birth defect or deprivation of oxygen at birth.*	The spine and brain. Work this area frequently during a treatment 6 or 7 times up and down each foot.
Cervical spondylosis	*Degenerative changes in the intervertebral discs in the cervical spine.*	The entire spine and chronic neck area.
Cholecystitis	*Inflammation of the gall bladder.*	Liver and gall bladder area.
Colic	*Waves of abdominal pain fluctuating in severity.*	Digestive system, solar plexus.
Colitis, diverticulitis and irritable bowel syndrome	*Inflammation of the colon.*	Entire digestive system and lumbar spine to help nerve and blood supply to the pelvic area.

Condition	Symptoms	Main area to treat
Conjunctivitis (eye condition)	*Inflammation of the conjunctiva.*	Eye/cervical spine and all sinus areas.
Constipation	*Difficulty in passing a motion.*	Entire intestines and liver/ gall bladder (bile helps lubrication of the bowel) and lumbar spinal nerves.
Crohn's disease	*Chronic form of enteritis affecting terminal parts of the ileum.*	Entire intestines and lumbar spine to help blood supply to pelvic area.
Cystitis	*Inflammation of the urinary system, mainly affecting the bladder.*	Urinary system. Coccyx, pelvis and lumbar spine.
Depression	*A feeling of gloom.*	Entire endocrine system to help balance hormonal output. Lots of work on relaxation techniques.
Diabetes	*Caused by a deficiency of insulin production of the pancreas.*	Digestive, endocrine, circulatory and respiratory systems and thoracic spine.
Down's syndrome		Cannot help condition but work respiratory system as this area is prone to illness.
Dysmenorrhoea	*Painful or difficult menstruation.*	Work urinary and reproductive, coccyx/ pelvis and lumbar spine.
Ear infection	*Infection and inflammation of the inner ear.*	Digestive system (mucus trying to eliminate), sinus, ear and eye.
Eczema and all skin diseases	*Inflammation of the skin.*	Treat as for asthma: comes from the same source. Digestive system and adrenals.

Condition	Symptoms	Main area to treat
Emphysema	*The over-distension of the lungs by air. Alveoli of the lungs distended due to atrophy of the alveolar walls.*	Treat as for asthma.
Endometriosis	*Inflammation of the endometrium.*	Reproductive and endocrine, can be a hormone imbalance.
Epilepsy	*Disorder of brain marked by the occurrence of convulsive fits.*	Brain and spine.
Fever	*A rise in normal body temperature.*	Pituitary, hypothalamus, thyroid.
Fibroid	*A tumour composed of mixed muscular and fibrous tissue in uterus.*	Reproductive system.
Glandular fever	*Fever with enlargement and tenderness of the lymphatic glands.*	Lymphatic system.
Gout (excessive uric acid)	*Inflamed red area: usually toes, elbow and knee.*	Digestive system, liver and kidneys.
Haemorrhoids	*Varicose veins in rectum.*	Descending colon and rectum, pelvic and coccyx.
Hay fever	*Allergic rhinitis.*	Sinus, ear, eye, adrenal, digestive system.
Headache	*Pain in head.*	Entire spine, brain.
Hepatitis	*Inflammation of liver causing nausea, upper abdominal discomfort, jaundice, itching of skin.*	Liver, digestive system and adrenals.

Condition	Symptoms	Main area to treat
Hiatus hernia	*Acid reflux after eating: pain in stomach.*	Digestive system, stomach, solar plexus.
Hypertension	*High blood pressure.*	Circulatory, respiratory and kidney. **Do not** work on the adrenals when treating high blood pressure.
Hypotension	*Low blood pressure.*	As above, **but work** on adrenals to increase levels.
Incontinence	*Absence of voluntary control of the passing of urine or faeces.*	Urinary/intestinal, lumbar spine, coccyx, pelvis.
Indigestion (dyspepsia)	*Failure of the digestive processes.*	Digestive and intestinal areas.
Insomnia	*Inability to sleep.*	Spine, brain, (pituitary), respiratory, circulatory and general treatment.
Iritis	*Inflammation of eye.*	Eye, kidney, neck, (urinary problems affect the eyes).
Lumbago	*Painful condition of the lumbar muscles due to inflammation. May be caused by displaced invertebral disc.*	Coccyx, pelvis, lumbar spine.
Mastitis	*Inflammation of the breast.*	Breast, shoulder, endocrine system.
Mastoiditis	*Inflammation of the mastoid bone in the ear.*	Head, neck, ear, cervical spine.
Ménière's disease	*Attacks of vertigo, nausea, tinnitus and hearing loss.*	Ear, head, sinuses, cervical spine and chronic neck.

Condition	Symptoms	Main area to treat
Migraine	*Paroxysmal attacks of headache usually with nausea also preceded by disorders of vision.*	Head, cervical neck and cervical spine; liver: often digestive in origin and the liver is usually affected.
Multiple sclerosis	*Degeneration of the myeline sheath in nerves.*	Spine, brain.
Myocarditis	*Inflammation of the myocardium.*	Respiratory, circulatory and thoracic spine.
Nephritis	*Inflammation of kidney.*	Urinary system, lumbar spine.
Neuralgia	*Pain in the nerves of face.*	First 3 toes, eye, ear, facial area, sinuses, cervical spine.
Oedema	*Abnormal amount of fluid in the tissues causing swelling, particularly in the ankles and legs.*	Urinary and circulatory systems, lumbar spine, lymphatic area surrounding groin.
Orchitis	*Inflammation of testicles.*	Reproductive, coccyx, pelvis, lumbar spine.
Osteoarthritis	*Disorder due to excessive wear and tear to joint surfaces affecting mainly weight-bearing joints, hips, knees and spine.*	Work out thoroughly prime joint or part of body affected, spine and urinary system to encourage good elimination.
Ovarian cysts	*Hormonal imbalance. Abdominal discomfort.*	Reproductive, endocrine. spine.
Palpitations	*Racing heart and anxiety.*	Chest, heart, solar plexus.
Pancreatitis	*Inflammation of pancreas.*	Digestive system.
Parkinson's disease	*Shaking of limbs, fixed, staring expression, poor coordination.*	Central nervous system, spine and brain.

Condition	Symptoms	Main area to treat
Phlebitis	*Inflammation of the veins.*	Circulatory, respiratory.
Pleurisy	*See Bronchitis and Asthma.*	
PMT	*Mood swings, bloating, swollen hands, depression, food binges.*	Endocrine, also reproductive systems.
Prostatis	*Prostate inflammation.*	Urinary and reproductive, also lumbar spine.
Quinsy	*Infected area in throat.*	Ear, throat, all toes, pituitary/hypothalamus.
Rheumatoid arthritis	*Pain, stiffness, swelling in joints eg knee, foot, hand, elbow, shoulder.*	Digestive, hip, pelvis, spine, elbow, shoulder, knee, thyroid/parathyroid.
Rhinitis or hay fever	*Inflammation of nose.*	Sinuses, nose/throat, adrenals to reduce inflammation, digestive system (often a food allergy).
Salpingitis	*Inflammation of fallopian tubes.*	Entire reproductive and endocrine systems plus coccyx. Pelvic/hip.
Sciatica	*Compression of the sciatic nerve causing pain.*	Lumbar spine, coccyx, pelvic/hip, sciatic area.
Shingles	*Inflammation of nerve endings in spine.*	All spinal areas.
Sinusitis	*Inflammation of facial sinuses.*	Sinuses, eye/ear, cervical spine, facial area.

Condition	Symptoms	Main area to treat
Spondylitis (as in ankylosing spondylitis)	*Inflammation of a vertebra. Ossification of spinal ligaments with ankylosis of the cervical and sacro-iliac joints. Unknown origin occurring characteristically in young men.*	Entire skeletal system.
Tennis elbow	*Inflammation of bursa of joint affecting the insertion of the extensor tendon of the forearm muscles.*	Cervical spine, shoulder, elbow.
Thrombosis (clot in circulatory system)	*Coagulation of blood in the vessels.*	Respiratory, circulatory systems, thoracic spine.
Thyrotoxicosis (Hyperthyroidism)	*Excess production of thyroxine.*	Thyroid and all endocrine glands.
Tinnitus	*Ringing in the ears.*	Neck, ear, sinuses, cervical spine.
Tonsillitis	*Inflammation of the tonsils.*	Throat, sinuses, cervical spine, thymus gland in young children to help immunity.
Trigeminal neuralgia	*Pains in the face of unknown cause.*	Face, sinuses, eye/ear, neck.
Urticaria	*An itchy rash caused by emotions or allergy.*	See asthma and eczema.
Varicose veins	*Caused by chronic constipation and pressure during pregnancy.*	Intestinal area, lumbar spine.
Vertigo	*Dizziness.*	Ear, head, sinuses, cervical spine.

CHAPTER 37 The treatment session

1   Make sure that the room that you are going to use to give your treatment session in is as comfortable as possible and away from noise which will disturb the treatment and make the possibility of relaxation difficult.

2   Display your Diploma of Reflexology, together with any certificates you may have showing membership to Associations, a First Aid Certificate, and a Certificate of Insurance on the wall of the room in which you are working. The public have the right to see when and where you were qualified; that you are a member of a recognised Association; that you are insured to practice and that you have attended a one day course in basic first aid and would, therefore, be able to handle competently and confidently any situation that could occur when treating the general public.

3   Some practitioners prefer to work from a Complementary Medical Centre, particularly if they have insufficient space in their own homes from which to practice. These Centres are fine, providing you have a sufficient number of patients to treat, as you will either have to pay a daily rental rate, or give the Centre a percentage of the fee for each treatment session. A daily rate therefore would prove to be very expensive if you only had three or four patients to see in any one day.

4   Home visits are becoming popular, particularly when treating the elderly who, because of disabilities, are not able to travel to you. Many practitioners are now obtaining work in Private Nursing Homes. Their attendance on a weekly basis to the elderly is very welcomed, not only in easing aches and pains, but in giving an elderly person an hour of your time – time not just to treat but to chat and listen. Communication alone is a wonderful healer.

5   Do dress as professionally as possible: trousers and a white tunic look smart, or you may prefer some other form of dress, but it is important to look clean and tidy. Do not wear bracelets, jangling earrings or rings with large stones.

6   Make sure that your hands and finger nails are well manicured, your hands are the tools of your trade!

7   **Taking a case history** You need to take as much information from your patients as possible in order to obtain good insight into their lifestyles and medical history. The taking of a detailed case history does give you a very clear picture of the person that you are about to treat.

Obvious details are: their age, type of employment (if this is applicable), whether they are married or single, whether they sleep well, what type of diet do they eat, do they smoke, drink, and if so approximately how much alcohol is consumed in any one week? In the case of young married people: how many children have they, are there any family histories of diseases or allergies? Are they on medication? Have they had surgery? Have they been involved in any accidents?

8   You need to allow about one hour for each patient; this gives you just a few minutes between patients in which to wash your hands, have a drink and prepare for the next appointment. It also leaves just a few minutes spare in case your patient happens to be late! The very worst thing you can do is to rush through a treatment: it takes away the whole principle of reflexology, which is a relaxing therapy.

9   It is important to place your patient in as comfortable a position as possible. Therefore, the use of a reclining chair, or a portable footstool known as a PorTa-Ped™ should be available. The PorTa-Ped™ is ideal for home visiting and if at any time you feel able to give a lecture where a demonstration will be needed, the PorTa-Ped™ is light and easy to carry about. However for every-day use a reclining chair really allows your patient to stretch out and relax with the legs in an elevated position and enjoy an hour of blissful relaxation.

10   Make sure you are sitting in a comfortable, relaxed position, and a therapist's adjustable stool which has five wheels and allows the therapist to rotate with ease from the right foot to the left is recommended.

11   Some pleasant, relaxing music in the background will enhance the mood and maybe even an oil burner, sending out a fragrant aroma in the treatment room, to really spoil your patients!

12   Do not use oils or creams. An oily foot makes it very difficult to isolate the reflex points. A very light dusting of baby powder is all that is needed.

13   Cover the legs of your patient with a large towel, and commence working on the right foot in the following manner.

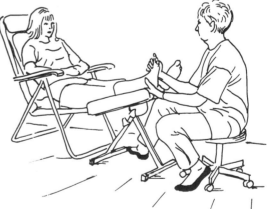

'Make sure you are sitting in a comfortable position: a therapist's adjustable stool is recommended and a reclining chair for your patient.'

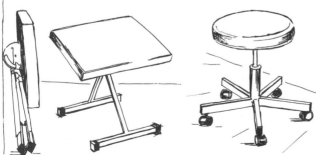

The PorTa-Ped™ and therapist's adjustable stool

Starting treatment

Note Figure references refer to the diagrams used throughout this book. The diagrams are repeated here as an aide-memoire.

Treatment record card
Record patient details and medical history.

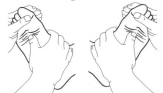

- Begin with the **Side-to-side relaxation exercise** on the right foot and repeat this on the left foot. *See Figures 5.5 and 5.6.*

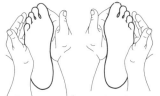

- Now use the **Diaphragm relaxation exercise.** Work on the right foot first and then the left. *See Figures 5.7 and 5.8.*

- This helps to relax the feet and body of your patient and in particular this exercise slows down the respiratory rate creating a sense of peace, very similar to the experience you have when you are 'just dropping off to sleep'.

THE RIGHT FOOT
Order of treatment

1 Work up the plantar side of the lung (remember to work from medial to lateral then lateral to medial. *See Figures 9.2 and 9.3.*

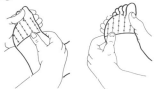

2 Work down the dorsal side of the lung/breast area. *See Figures 9.4 and 9.5.*

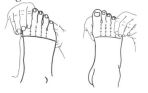

3 Use the **Metartarsal kneading exercise.** *See Figures 5.9 and 5.10.*

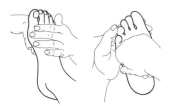

4 Work up all the toe areas. (You will be working out both the endocrine area in the brain as well as the sinuses.) *See Figures 19.2 and 19.3.*

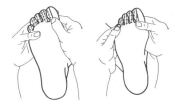

5 Work out the eye and ear using the rotating method. *See Figures 19.6 and 19.7.*

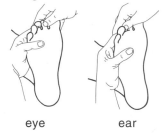

eye   ear

6 Work out the neck/thyroid (plantar side). *See Figure 14.4.*

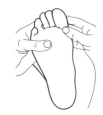

7 Work out the neck/thyroid (dorsal side). *See Figure 14.5.*

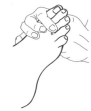

8 Work out the coccyx, pelvis and hip. *See Figures 21.4 and 21.5.*

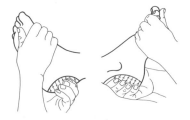

9 Work up the spine over the brain. (Working out the skeletal system simultaneously works the central nervous system. *See Figures 21.6 and 21.7.*

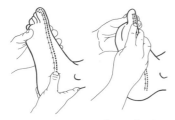

10 Work out the chronic neck. *See Figure 21.9.*

11 Work out the front of the face. *See Figure 19.10.*

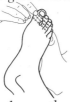

12 Work down the spine. *See Figure 21.8.*

13 Work out the shoulder area. *See Figures 21.10 and 21.11.*

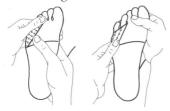

14 Work out the knee/elbow area. *See Figure 21.12.*

15 Work out the primary sciatic area. *See Figure 21.13.*

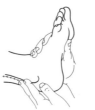

16 Work out the secondary sciatic area. *See Figure 21.14.*

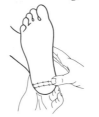

17 Work out the liver area. *See Figures 7.2. and 7.3.*

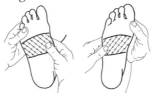

18 Use the hooking out technique on the ileo-caecal valve. *See Figure 7.6.*

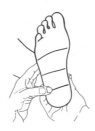

19 Work out the entire intestinal area to the base of the heel. (This includes the buttock and back of the pelvic area.) *See Figures 7.7. and 7.8.*

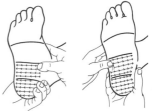

20 Use the **Ankle freeing exercise**. *See Figure 5.13.*

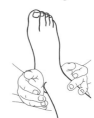

21 Work out the bladder, ureter tube to kidney. *See Figure 23.2.*

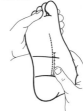

22 Use both the **Undergrip and Overgrip relaxation exercises**. *See Figures 5.15 and 5.19.*

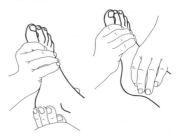

23 Work out the area of the uterus/prostate. *See Figures 25.2 and 25.3.*

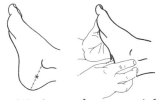

24 Work out the area of the ovary/testicle. *See Figure 25.4.*

25 Work out the fallopian tube/vas deferens. *See Figure 25.5.*

27 Use the **Foot moulding relaxation exercise.** *See Figures 5.21 and 5.22.*

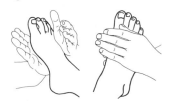

28 Use the **Rib cage relaxation exercise.** *See Figures 5.25 and 5.26.*

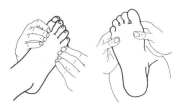

Treatment record card

• At this stage record the sensitivities found on the right foot on your patient's Treatment Record.

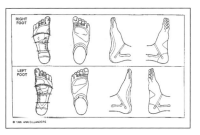

• It is recommended that you colour in the area that is revealing a sensitivity with a red pen. This card then acts almost like an X-ray showing how internal congestions, inflammations and irritations reflect as a sensitivity in the reflexes in the feet.

THE LEFT FOOT

• You have already worked on the left foot with the Side-to-side relaxation exercise and Diaphragm relaxation exercise when you began the treatment, so there is no need to work over that area again.

• Remember, the reflexes on the left foot are not identical to the right, because we have certain organs on the left foot which we do not have on the right, such as the heart, the stomach, the pancreas, and the spleen.

THE LEFT FOOT
Order of treatment

1 Work up the plantar side of the lung. *See Figures 9.6 and 9.7.*

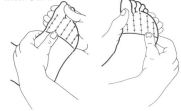

2 Work down the dorsal side of the lung/breast area. *See Figures 9.8 and 9.9.*

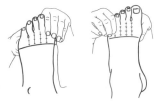

3 Work out the heart area. *See Figure 11.2.*

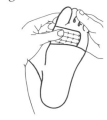

4 Use the **Metatarsal kneading relaxation exercise.** *See Figures 5.11 and 5.12.*

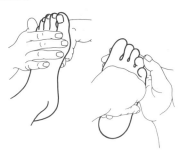

5 Work all the areas relating to the toes, remember, these are the sinus areas as well as the pituitary gland which is in the medial side of the big toe. Make sure you cover the entire surface area of these toes. *See Figures 19.4 and 19.5.*

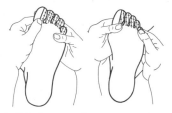

6 Work out the eye and ear reflex using the rotation technique. *See Figures 19.8 and 19.9.*

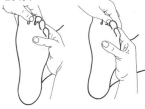

eye   ear

7 Work on the neck/thyroid (plantar side first). *See Figure 14.6.*

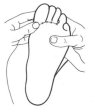

8 Work out the neck/thyroid (dorsal side). *See Figure 14.7.*

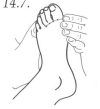

9 Work on the coccyx, then pelvis and hip. *See Figures 21.15 and 21.16.*

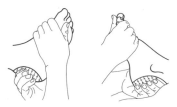

10 Work up the spine over the brain. *See Figures 21.17 and 21.18.*

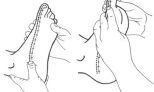

11 Work the chronic neck area. *See Figure 21.20.*

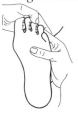

12 Work the front of the face. *See Figure 19.11.*

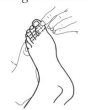

13 Work down the spine. *See Figure 21.19.*

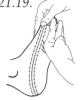

14 Work out the shoulder area. *See Figures 21.21 and 21.22.*

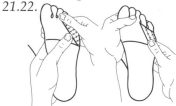

15 Work out the knee/elbow area. *See Figure 21.23.*

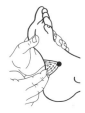

16 Work out the primary sciatic area. *See Figure 21.24.*

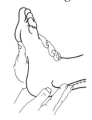

17 Work out the secondary sciatic area. *See Figure 21.25.*

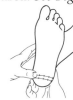

18 Work out the stomach, pancreas and spleen. *See Figures 7.4 and 7.5.*

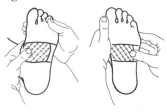

19 Work out the transverse, and descending colon. *See Figures 7.9 and 7.10.*

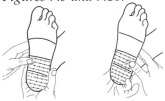

20 Work out the sigmoid colon. *See Figure 7.11.*

21 Use the **Ankle freeing relaxation exercise.** *See Figure 5.14.*

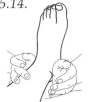

22 Work out the bladder, ureter tube to kidney. *See Figure 23.4.*

23 Use both the **Undergrip and Overgrip relaxation exercises.** *See Figures 5.16 and 5.20*

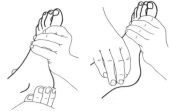

24 Work out the area of the uterus/prostate. *See Figures 25.6 and 25.7.*

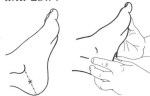

25 Work out the area of the ovary/testicle. *See Figure 25.8.*

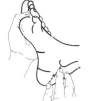

26 Work out the fallopian tube/vas deferens. *See Figure 25.9.*

27 Use the **Foot moulding relaxation exercise.** *See Figures 5.23 and 5.24.*

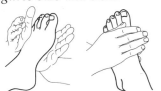

28 Use the **Rib cage relaxation exercise.** *See Figures 5.27 and 5.28.*

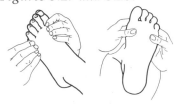

• Record at this stage the sensitivities found on the left foot.

• Return to the right foot and just work over the sensitivities on the right foot two or three times.

• Repeat the same procedure on the left foot.

• You should find that the sensitivities have already decreased which means that you have effected a good treatment session.

• You should aim to complete your treatment within one hour.

• Most patients get a good result from reflexology treatments within six sessions. The more chronic states tend to take a little more time.

• As soon as the ache or pain or symptom abates, lengthen the gap between treatments and see your patient in a fortnight. If all is well within two weeks, then ask the patient to return in a month, just to make sure that the condition does not return.

• It would be in the interest of the patient, particularly if the condition is chronic and long standing, to have periodic treatments, say once in six weeks, just to enable the body to maintain its new found health and vitality.

However, the decision for regular treatments does ultimately rest with the patient.

• **Just one warning** – if a patient presents with a painful condition that has not been diagnosed by the doctor, and they too are unaware of the actual cause, do not continue with more than four treatments. If you are not getting a good result, it could mean that there is a deep seated problem that needs investigating.

• Reflexologists are not doctors: they do not have access to X-rays, scanning machines and blood tests to help with reaching a satisfactory conclusion for the cause of the symptoms.

'An attractive treatment room with patient relaxing in a comfortable, reclining chair –The Vita-Standard Adjustable Chair. Treatment equipment is available from The British School of Reflexology - 01279 445234.'

CHAPTER 38 We are what we eat

For many thousands of years the human race has managed without any technical knowledge of nutrition. Man relied on his instinct and was certainly more in touch with his feelings. When illness occurred he knew exactly what to do to restore himself to health and harmony.

In the many ancient healing traditions of the Native American, the Egyptians, and Chinese the elements for health and vitality were herbs, water, sunlight, fresh air, simple whole foods and sleep and it is interesting to note that we are the only 'human animal' on this planet that ever suffers from insomnia!

Disease was regarded as a disharmony of the body mind and spirit and consequently, in order for harmony to be restored, these three elements needed to be looked at. When illness came restoration of health was achieved by the healing power of nature and the self healing of the body – this unity is referred to as naturopathy and is as old as life itself.

Hippocrates (460-377 BC), the Father of naturopathic medicine, believed that only nature heals, but the conditions must be right in the body for healing to take place.

Fasting is one of the prime examples of restoring the body back to harmony and was used extensively by many civilisations, and still is to-day, although not as extensively as it might. Most people still feel that if they do not receive their three meals a day they will expire rapidly.

What do animals do when they are sick? They curl up in a ball, make sure that sufficient water is available and eat nothing. It is impossible to make a sick animal eat; they just utterly refuse to even open their mouths. They still have this inbuilt knowledge of how their body needs to be treated when sick.

Fasting is effective because it gives the entire system a rest and an opportunity to eliminate waste without the need to digest food, which takes up body energy.

What you can do to improve your diet

• Reduce your refined sugar. Sugar is a useless food and is actually bad for us.

• Salt and caffeine intake should be reduced to a minimum.

• Try to eat food that is as uncontaminated as possible.

• Eat only when you are hungry and chew your food thoroughly.

• Increase your intake of pure spring water. Most of us do not drink enough pure fluid. Try to have herbal teas if you do not like just pure cold water: there are so many different varieties to try.

• Eat some raw salad and at least four pieces of fresh fruit daily.

• Make sure you are getting sufficient dietary fibre. Only have break-fast cereals that have no added sugar.

The life force can concentrate all its efforts on healing and that is exactly how healing was encouraged.

A three day fast is sufficient to restore the average person back to health. As you fast, your body rapidly eliminates all the waste, and provided sufficient fluid is taken you can, if you wish, have diluted grape or apple juice, or diluted vegetable juices if this is preferable and your body will detoxify.

Hippocrates had such strong, sensible foundations of knowledge of how to achieve good health and also how to attract disease.

He said, 'Whosoever shall eat or drink more or less than he should, or shall sleep more or less, or shall labour more or less from idleness or from hardship, without doubt, he will not escape sickness.'

These conditions are no longer respected in modern medicine to-day. The patient looks to his doctor to heal him of his dilemma; a bottle of pills; surgery. Few people change the conditions that caused the disease in the first place and put that right; that is why their illnesses become chronic.

Cutting out a tumour or giving a patient with a heart condition a bypass operation does not ultimately 'heal'; it improves the health of the patient temporarily, but if the reason for the condition is not changed, then more disease will ultimately rear its ugly head once again.

By the 18th century the relationship between food and disease had been forgotton as treatments such as bleeding, often by the help of leeches, and highly toxic medicines containing antimony and mercury came into being.

After the first World War pharmocologists began to look forward to the time when there would be 'a pill for every ill' when artifical drugs would be able to produce any desired effect on the body. The gentle treatments such as fasting, the use of plants and vegetables to heal, proper breathing, moderations of living, acupuncture and osteopathy were buried.

Since the mid 1940s all natural therapies have gone completely out of fashion as a 'rapid recovery' is the order of the day for the patient and doctor, with the use of synthetically produced drugs for every ill which causes

What you can do to improve your diet

• Do not buy products that contain lists of E additives, flavourings and colourings. Read the back of each packet and jar before you buy.

• The popular white loaf may contain an excess of bleaching agents and chalk and have additives a yard long, in order to keep it fresher for longer, and whiter than white. In our digestive systems it just clogs our bowel, rather like balls of cotton wool. White bread, and white sugar are one of the causative factors for the increase in bowel cancer.

• Eating for health is eating what you should instinctively know is best for you and do not be taken in by what the advertisers brainwash you into believing you need.

a toxic chemical factory within the human body.

However, within the last ten years a revolution is occurring as more people become disenchanted with drugs and the unpleasant side effects which are often far worse than the illness that is being treated.

All forms of complementary medicines are becoming so popular, with interest in diet reforms, massage, aromatherapy, acupuncture, shiatsu and reflexology, to name but a few.

The gentle art of healing is returning, but there is not sufficient respect from the medical profession when patients make such efforts in trying to heal themselves. They are looked upon as 'bad parents' if they refuse immunisation for their children, but it is now a well known fact that vaccinations and immunisations are responsible for so many disorders of the body and mind: autism, and dyslexia, plus the huge increase in 'learning and behavioural' problems – many of these problems have been linked to vaccination.

The whooping cough vaccine has been linked to the increase of asthma in children. Yes, you may say, but many children died of whooping cough. Many children die from the effects of an asthmatic attack, too!

Sufferers from cancer, the brave ones, who have refused all invasive treatments such as chemotherapy and radiotherapy and chosen to try a different approach, have been instilled with fear by the medical profession, as to what will happen if they do not allow the conventional treatments for cancer to be used on them.

The treatment for cancer, in the main, is crude and not very effective. Some people do survive the treatments but many, unfortunately, do not. However, many have proved the doctors wrong as they seek another solution for their disease: they take the responsibility for their illness into their own hands. These people are to be so admired, and many of them have gone on to live for years with changes in diet, lifestyle, vitamin and mineral supplementation and treating their bodies 'kindly'.

When we eat huge, fatty, fried meals, indulge in plates of chips, give our toddlers cans of coke and highly coloured sugar and saccharin laced drinks plus bags of crisps and a huge consumption of sweets, we are actually subjecting ourselves and our children to internal abuse. We are willingly harming their bodies with destructive substances. Most parents would be alarmed at this statement and would be horrified if anybody abused their children physically, but really there is little difference.

Your child will suffer greatly from pain and discomfort in their early years if they have repeated attacks of ear, nose and throat infections, bronchitis, and asthma. Many of these maladies can be removed by attention to nutrition and health style.

Cow's milk contains far too much protein which places an undue stress on a baby's kidneys, which in turn are unable to fulfil their eliminating functions efficiently.

In most Western countries the amount of money spent by governments on promoting healthy diets, healthy lives and an understanding of the laws of nature is less than one fortieth of the money spent by the Food Industry, who spend millions every year in trying to get the public to eat a new type of chocolate bar; a bag of new flavoured crisps; bigger and better pizzas; the newest alcoholic beverage.

It is strange how those who advertise these products are always so slim, fit looking and beautiful. We do not see the obese male with an enormous beer belly caused by excessive eating and drinking; or the obese female who waddles to the supermarket and walks breathlessly up and down the ailes where a never-ending selection of foods confronts her; or the wheezy toddler whose mother believes that a large milk consumption is essential for the health of her child even though his wheezy chest and frequent bronchitic attacks may well be an inability of his digestive system to cope with cow's milk!

'The doctor of the future will give no medicine, but will interest his patient in the care of the human frame, in diet and in the cause and prevention of disease.'
Thomas Eddison.

Conclusion

We are entering into a new millineum; into a new awareness of the holistic approach to illness; into a new age which hopefully will teach man that the destruction of this wonderful planet was due to him. It was he who produced wars in attempts to gain power, money and enforce his will on others.

The destruction of the rain forests was manmade; the pollution of our seas and rivers was his responsibility too.

The mindless extinction of the dolphins and wales and the cruel processes of farming animals who are cooped up in areas where any form of movement is a luxury and subsequent transportation abroad, leaves much to be desired. The insensitive destruction of animals in our slaughter-houses needs more control and a change in the attitudes of those involved.

It is pointless looking up into the heavens and asking our God – whoever each proposes him to be – to change the world and bring peace and harmony.

There is only one way that the peace of the world will ever be restored and that is when each one of us works at achieving peace and harmony at first with our families, friends and neighbours. We will then need to make every effort to preserve our planet rather than to abuse and spoil.

There really is only one natural system for healing the body and that is to abide by the laws of Nature.

INDEX

An *ITALICS* entry indicates an anatomy and physiology diagram. A **BOLD** entry indicates a Practical Procedure illustration. All other entries indicate text references.

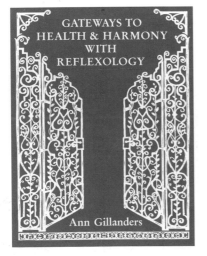

GATEWAYS TO HEALTH & HARMONY
WITH REFLEXOLOGY
(ISBN 0-9511868-4-1)
is a companion book to this title and contains
detailed Case Histories.
Available from
The British School of Reflexology:
Telephone 01279 429060
Fax 01279 445234